NO GALLBLADDER DIET COOKBOOK

'COMFORT DIGEST FORMULA'

Banish Mealtime Discomfort with Proven and Bloat-Busting Recipes Designed to Support Your Digestive Wellness

28-Day Gut-Soothing Meal Plan

ADA BENNETT

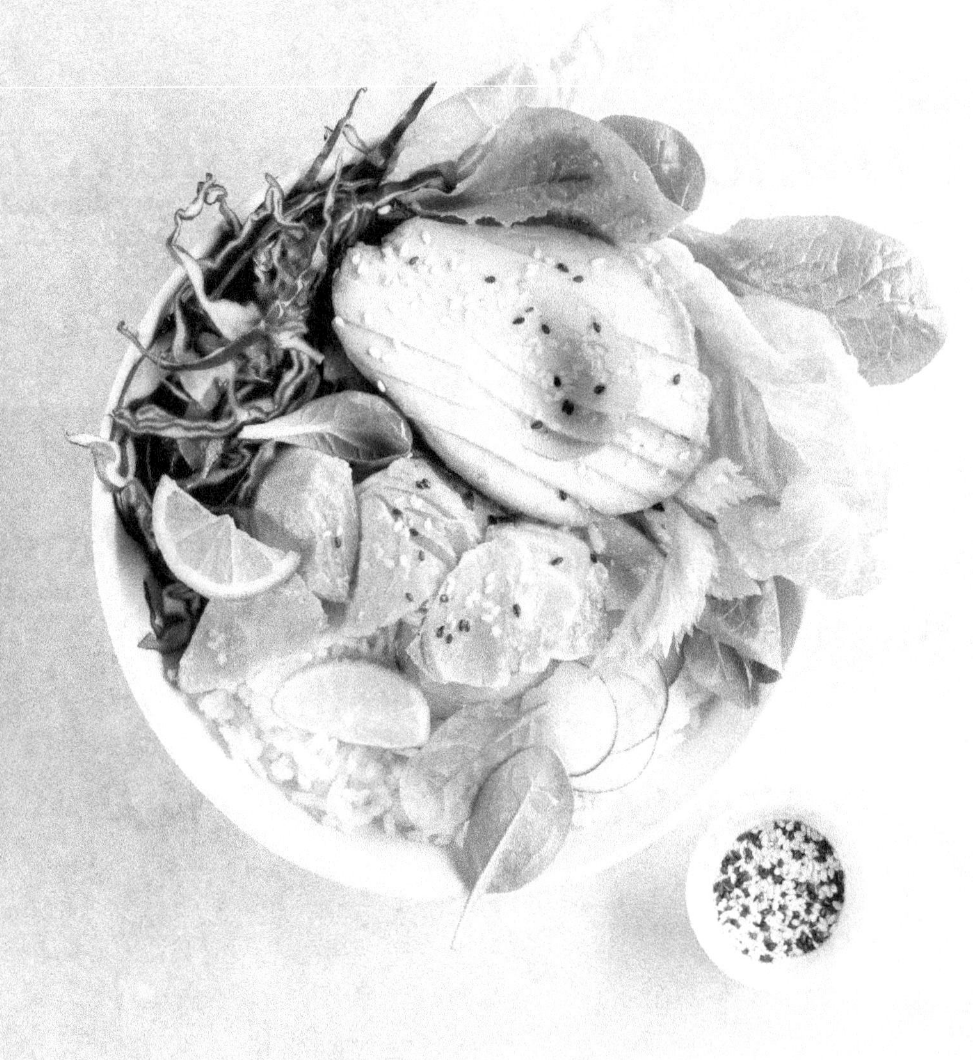

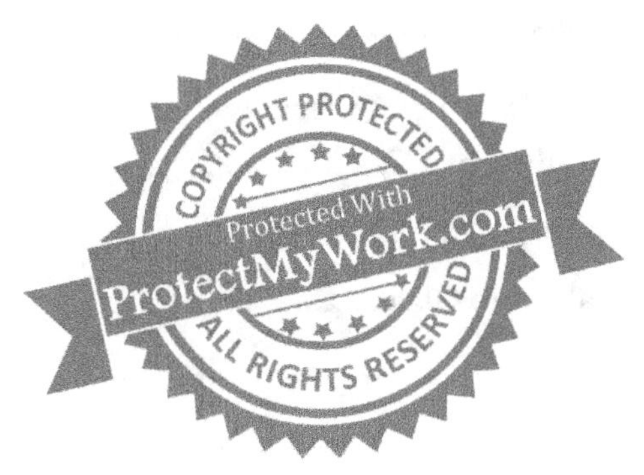
COPYRIGHT PROTECTED
Protected With
ProtectMyWork.com
ALL RIGHTS RESERVED

Table of Contents:

Introduction

Welcome to Your New Journey

Welcome to your new path forward after gallbladder removal—a practical guide tailored to your dietary needs. Removing your gallbladder can bring about significant changes in how you process food, and adjusting to these changes is crucial. This book is crafted to help you manage your diet efficiently, providing clear, actionable advice to ease this transition. Here, you'll learn how to enjoy your meals confidently, ensuring they support your health without causing discomfort. Let's begin this straightforward journey to better understanding and managing your post-gallbladder diet.

Understanding Your Gallbladder-Free Body

When your gallbladder is removed, your body's method of digesting fats undergoes a significant adjustment. Typically, the gallbladder stores bile from the liver, releasing it in response to fat intake to aid digestion. Without this reservoir, bile trickles continuously into your intestines, often not synchronizing with meal times. This mismatch can lead to difficulties in breaking down fatty foods, causing symptoms like bloating and indigestion. To manage these changes, it's important to modify your diet. By focusing on lower-fat meals and incorporating foods that are easier to digest, you can help your body adapt to its new digestive process and reduce discomfort. Additionally, spreading out your fat intake throughout the day can align better with the constant flow of bile, helping to ensure more effective fat digestion and overall comfort.

The Power of Food: Managing Your Diet for Comfort and Joy

Food has a powerful role in both our physical health and emotional well-being, especially when navigating life without a gallbladder. Tailoring your diet to suit this new reality is not just about avoiding discomfort; it's also about rediscovering enjoyment in eating. A carefully planned gallbladder-free diet helps prevent common digestive issues like bloating and indigestion, which can significantly enhance your physical comfort. Additionally, knowing which foods to choose and how to prepare them restores a sense of control and pleasure in eating. This not only improves your quality of life but also supports your emotional health by reducing food-related stress and anxiety. By embracing this tailored approach, you can enjoy meals that are both nourishing and satisfying, ensuring that each dish contributes positively to your overall well-being.

Part I: Building Your No Gallbladder Diet Foundation

Nutritional Guidelines for a Gallbladder-Free Lifestyle

Adapting to a gallbladder-free lifestyle necessitates a nuanced understanding of nutritional balance, particularly concerning macronutrients and micronutrients. The key is to optimize the intake of fats, proteins, and carbohydrates to support your altered digestive capabilities. Without a gallbladder, managing fat intake becomes crucial as your body can no longer store bile to release in response to heavy meals. Opt for moderate amounts of healthy fats like avocados, olive oil, and nuts, which are essential but easier on digestion when consumed in appropriate portions.

Proteins and carbohydrates remain vital, providing energy and supporting overall health without straining the digestive system. Include lean protein sources such as poultry, fish, legumes, and tofu, and favor complex carbohydrates like whole grains, fruits, and vegetables to ensure a steady energy supply and maintain blood sugar levels.

Micronutrients also demand attention, particularly fat-soluble vitamins (A, D, E, K), which may be harder to absorb post-gallbladder removal. Including sources of these vitamins in your diet, alongside foods rich in dietary fiber to aid in their absorption, ensures you do not miss out on these crucial nutrients. Balancing these elements in your daily meals not only helps in managing your physical health but also contributes to a feeling of well-being, enabling you to lead a full and active life despite the absence of your gallbladder.

Foods to Embrace and Foods to Avoid

Navigating your diet without a gallbladder means becoming familiar with which foods to embrace for comfort and health, and which to avoid to prevent discomfort and digestive issues. Here's a comprehensive guide to help you make informed choices:

Foods to Embrace:

1. **Lean Proteins:** Chicken, turkey, fish, and plant-based proteins like lentils and beans are easier on your digestion and provide essential nutrients without overloading your system with fats.
2. **Whole Grains:** Foods like brown rice, oats, quinoa, and whole wheat provide fiber that helps regulate digestion and prevent constipation.
3. **Low-Fat Dairy Alternatives:** Opt for low-fat or fat-free dairy options like milk, yogurt, and cheese to reduce fat intake while still getting your calcium and vitamin D.

4. **Fruits and Vegetables:** A staple in any healthy diet, fruits and vegetables are rich in vitamins, minerals, and fibers. Focus on non-cruciferous options to minimize gas, such as bell peppers, carrots, cucumbers, and berries.

5. **Healthy Fats:** While excessive fats are to be avoided, healthy fats from avocados, olive oil, and small portions of nuts and seeds are important for your overall health.

Foods to Avoid:

1. **Fatty Meats:** Avoid high-fat cuts of meat like pork, lamb, and the darker parts of chicken or turkey. These can stimulate bile production and may cause discomfort.

2. **Fried Foods:** These are typically high in unhealthy fats and can be very difficult to digest without a gallbladder, leading to pain and bloating.

3. **Spicy Foods:** Spices may irritate the digestive system and exacerbate symptoms like diarrhea and discomfort.

4. **Processed Foods:** High in fats and additives, processed foods can be hard on your digestion. Limit consumption of snacks, ready meals, and anything with artificial additives.

5. **High-Fat Dairy Products:** Rich dairy products such as cream, whole milk, and ice cream should be consumed sparingly as they can prompt symptoms of indigestion and discomfort.

By adhering to this guide and moderating your intake of certain foods, you can effectively manage your diet and minimize any digestive issues associated with living without a gallbladder. Remember, individual tolerance can vary, so it may be helpful to keep a food diary to track how different foods affect you personally. This will allow you to tailor your diet more precisely for optimal health and comfort. _To further enhance your dietary management, purchasers of the paperback version of this book will receive exclusive access to the **"Daily Digest Tracker"** This comprehensive journal helps you monitor what you eat and how your body reacts, allowing you to tailor your diet to your unique needs. Track your food intake, digestive responses, and personal adjustments to discover patterns and craft a personalized eating plan that minimizes discomfort and maximizes health benefits._

Managing Fat Intake Without a Gallbladder

Managing fat intake without a gallbladder is crucial for maintaining comfort and health. Without the gallbladder's reservoir of bile to aid in fat digestion, it becomes important to moderate fat consumption to avoid digestive distress. Here are strategies for incorporating healthy fats into your diet while recognizing limits to ensure you stay comfortable and healthy:

Choose Healthy Fats: Focus on consuming fats that are easier to digest and beneficial for your overall health. Incorporate sources of monounsaturated and polyunsaturated fats, such as avocados, nuts, seeds, and olive oil. These fats are not only easier on your system but also essential for heart health and overall well-being.

Moderate Portion Sizes: Even healthy fats should be consumed in moderation. Use measuring spoons or a food scale to add healthy oils to your dishes, and be mindful of the portion sizes of nuts and seeds, which are high in fat.

Spread Out Fat Intake: Instead of consuming large amounts of fat in one meal, spread your fat intake throughout the day. This approach helps manage the continuous flow of bile into your intestines, making it easier to digest the fats without overwhelming your system.

Cook Smart: When cooking, opt for methods that require less fat. Baking, steaming, grilling, and sautéing with a small amount of oil can make meals easier to digest. Avoid deep-frying and sautéing with large quantities of fat, as these methods increase the fat content significantly.

Read Labels: Be vigilant about reading nutritional labels on packaged foods. This can help you avoid hidden fats often found in processed foods, which can be particularly challenging to digest without a gallbladder.

Listen to Your Body: Pay close attention to how your body responds to different types and amounts of fats. If certain fats cause discomfort, try reducing the amount or switching to lighter alternatives.

By implementing these strategies, you can effectively manage your fat intake, which is vital for avoiding discomfort and promoting a healthier, more balanced diet after gallbladder removal.

Part II: The Recipes

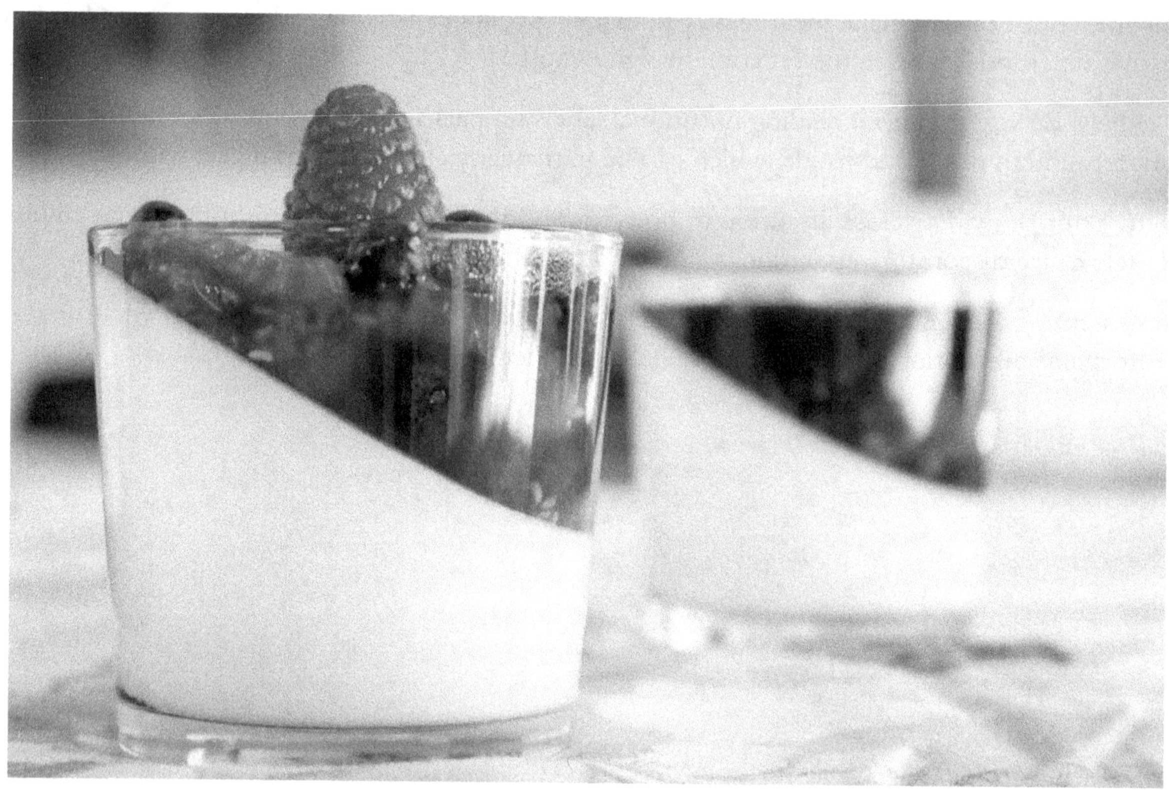

Low-Fat Blueberry Yogurt Parfait

Preparation Time: 10 minutes | Cooking Time: 0 minutes | Portion Size: 1 parfait | Difficulty Level: Easy

Ingredients:

- 1 cup low-fat Greek yogurt
- ½ cup fresh blueberries
- 2 tablespoons honey
- ¼ cup granola (low-fat, low-sugar)
- 1 tablespoon sliced almonds
- 1 tablespoon chia seeds
- 1 teaspoon vanilla extract

Instructions:

1. In a small bowl, mix the Greek yogurt with honey and vanilla extract until well combined.

2. In a parfait glass or a small bowl, layer ⅓ of the yogurt mixture at the bottom.

3. Add a layer of blueberries, granola, and sliced almonds.

4. Repeat the layering process twice more, finishing with a layer of granola and a sprinkle of chia seeds on top.

5. Serve immediately or refrigerate for up to 2 hours before serving.

Nutritional Information (per serving):

Total Carbohydrates: 38g | **Fiber:** 5g | **Sugars:** 20g | **Protein:** 14g | **Total Fat:** 7g | **Saturated Fat:** 1g | **Calories:** 285 | **Sodium:** 90mg | **Calcium:** 200mg | **Vitamin C:** 6mg | **Iron:** 2mg

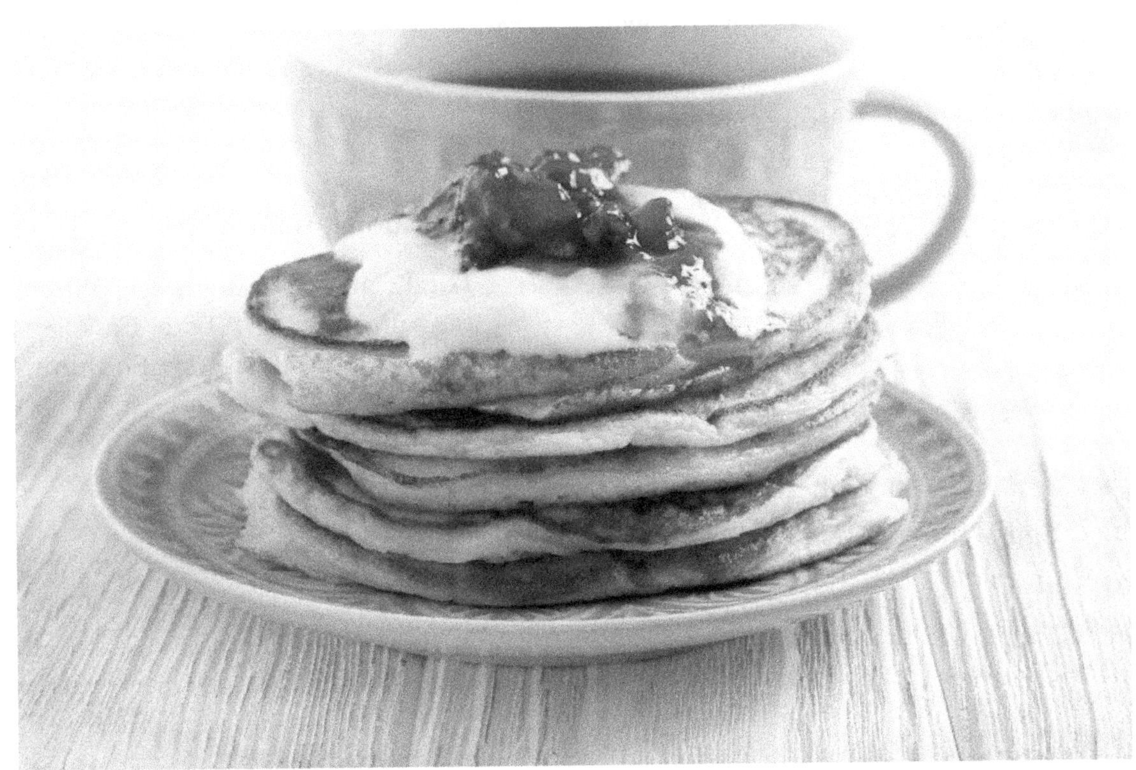

Oatmeal Pancakes with Fresh Strawberry Sauce

Preparation Time: 10 minutes | Cooking Time: 20 minutes | Portion Size: 4 pancakes | Difficulty Level: Easy

Ingredients:

Pancakes:

- 1 cup rolled oats
- 1 cup low-fat milk
- 1 large egg
- 1 teaspoon vanilla extract
- 1 tablespoon honey
- ½ teaspoon baking powder
- ¼ teaspoon salt
- Non-stick cooking spray

Strawberry Sauce:

- 1 cup fresh strawberries, hulled and sliced

- 1 tablespoon honey

- 1 teaspoon lemon juice

Instructions:

1. **Prepare the Pancakes:**

   1. In a blender, combine rolled oats, milk, egg, vanilla extract, honey, baking powder, and salt. Blend until smooth.

   2. Heat a non-stick skillet over medium heat and lightly coat with cooking spray.

   3. Pour ¼ cup of batter onto the skillet for each pancake. Cook until bubbles form on the surface and edges appear set, about 2-3 minutes. Flip and cook for another 1-2 minutes until golden brown.

   4. Transfer to a plate and repeat with remaining batter.

2. **Make the Fresh Strawberry Sauce:**

   1. In a small saucepan over medium heat, combine strawberries, honey, and lemon juice.

   2. Cook, stirring occasionally, until strawberries break down and sauce thickens, about 5-7 minutes.

   3. Remove from heat and let cool slightly.

3. **Serve:**

   1. Top pancakes with fresh strawberry sauce.

   2. Serve warm and enjoy!

Nutritional Information (per serving):

Total Carbohydrates: 42g | **Fiber:** 4g | **Sugars:** 16g | **Protein:** 8g | **Total Fat:** 3g | **Saturated Fat:** 1g | **Calories:** 215 | **Sodium:** 280mg | **Calcium:** 120mg | **Iron:** 1mg

Scrambled Egg Whites with Spinach and Mushrooms

Preparation Time: 5 minutes | Cooking Time: 10 minutes | Portion Size: 2 servings | Difficulty Level: Easy

Ingredients:

- 4 large egg whites

- 1 cup fresh spinach, chopped

- ½ cup mushrooms, sliced

- ¼ cup low-fat feta cheese, crumbled

- 2 tablespoons low-fat milk

- 1 tablespoon olive oil

- Salt and pepper to taste

Instructions:

1. In a small bowl, whisk together the egg whites and milk until well combined. Season with salt and pepper.

2. Heat olive oil in a non-stick skillet over medium heat. Add mushrooms and sauté until softened, about 3-4 minutes.

3. Add the spinach to the skillet and cook for another 1-2 minutes until wilted.

4. Pour the egg white mixture into the skillet, stirring gently with a spatula. Cook until eggs are just set but still soft, about 2-3 minutes.

5. Remove from heat and sprinkle with crumbled feta cheese.

6. Serve immediately and enjoy!

Nutritional Information (per serving):

Total Carbohydrates: 4g | **Fiber:** 1g | **Sugars:** 2g | **Protein:** 14g | **Total Fat:** 8g | **Saturated Fat:** 2g | **Calories:** 130 | **Sodium:** 180mg |

Calcium: 100mg | **Iron:** 2mg | **Vitamin B12:** 0.4mcg

Banana Almond Smoothie Bowl

Preparation Time: 10 minutes | Cooking Time: 0 minutes | Portion Size: 1 bowl | Difficulty Level: Easy

Ingredients:

- 1 frozen banana, sliced
- ½ cup unsweetened almond milk
- 2 tablespoons almond butter
- 1 tablespoon chia seeds
- 1 teaspoon vanilla extract
- ¼ cup granola (low-fat, low-sugar)
- 2 tablespoons sliced almonds
- Fresh berries (e.g., blueberries, strawberries) for topping

Instructions:

1. In a blender, combine frozen banana, almond milk, almond butter, chia seeds, and vanilla extract. Blend until smooth and creamy.

2. Pour the smoothie into a bowl.

3. Top with granola, sliced almonds, and fresh berries.

4. Serve immediately and enjoy!

Nutritional Information (per serving):

Total Carbohydrates: 45g | **Fiber:** 8g | **Sugars:** 20g | **Protein:** 10g | **Total Fat:** 15g | **Saturated Fat:** 2g | **Calories:** 320 | **Sodium:** 120mg | **Calcium:** 180mg | **Iron:** 2mg | **Vitamin B12:** 0.2mcg

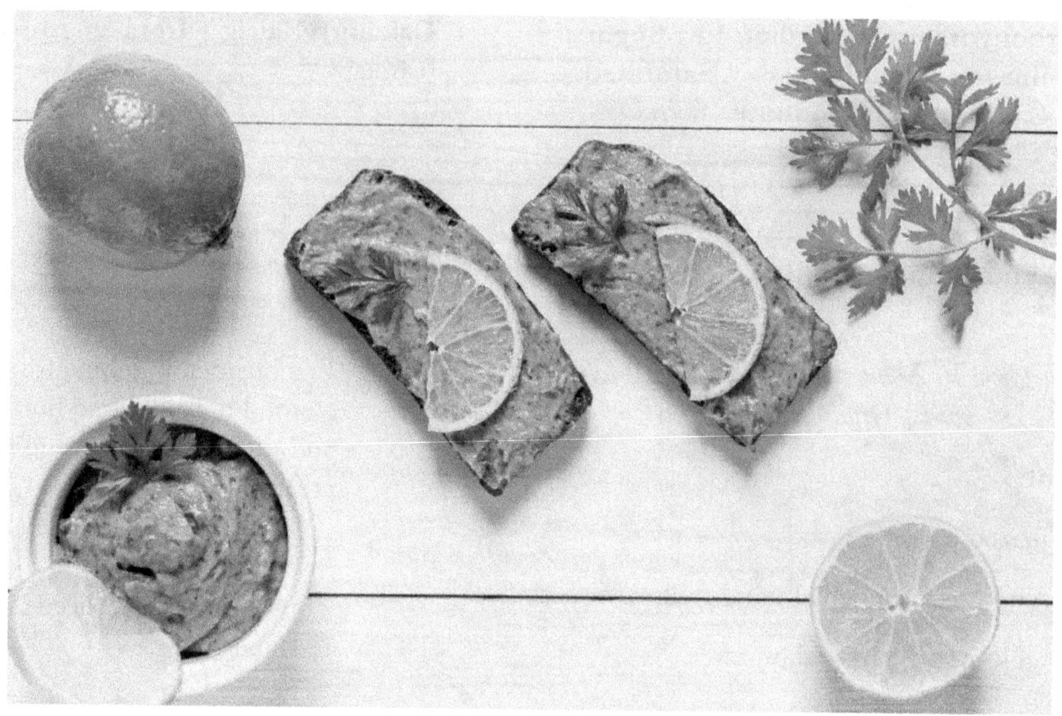

Avocado Toast on Whole Grain Bread

Preparation Time: 5 minutes | Cooking Time: 5 minutes | Portion Size: 2 servings | Difficulty Level: Easy

Ingredients:

- 2 slices whole grain bread
- 1 ripe avocado, peeled and pitted
- 1 teaspoon lemon juice
- 1 tablespoon olive oil
- Salt and pepper to taste
- 1 tablespoon chopped fresh cilantro
- 1 tablespoon pumpkin seeds (optional)

Instructions:

1. Toast the slices of whole grain bread to your desired level of crispness.

2. In a small bowl, mash the avocado with a fork. Add lemon juice, olive oil, salt, and pepper, and mix until smooth.

3. Spread the avocado mixture evenly on the toasted bread slices.

4. Sprinkle with chopped cilantro and pumpkin seeds if desired.

5. Serve immediately and enjoy!

Nutritional Information (per serving):

Total Carbohydrates: 23g | **Fiber:** 7g | **Sugars:** 2g | **Protein:** 4g | **Total Fat:** 17g | **Saturated Fat:** 3g | **Calories:** 230 | **Sodium:** 150mg | **Calcium:** 30mg | **Iron:** 1.5mg | **Vitamin C:** 8mg

Turkey Bacon and Egg White Muffins

Preparation Time: 10 minutes | Cooking Time: 20 minutes | Portion Size: 12 muffins | Difficulty Level: Easy

Ingredients:

- 6 slices turkey bacon, cooked and crumbled
- 2 cups egg whites
- ½ cup low-fat cheddar cheese, shredded
- ¼ cup red bell pepper, diced
- ¼ cup green onion, chopped
- ½ teaspoon salt
- ¼ teaspoon black pepper
- Non-stick cooking spray

Instructions:

1. Preheat the oven to 350°F (180°C). Spray a muffin tin with non-stick cooking spray.
2. In a large bowl, whisk together egg whites, cheddar cheese, bell pepper, green onion, salt, and black pepper.
3. Divide the crumbled turkey bacon evenly among the 12 muffin cups.
4. Pour the egg white mixture over the turkey bacon, filling each muffin cup about three-quarters full.
5. Bake for 18-20 minutes or until the egg muffins are set and lightly browned.
6. Allow to cool slightly before removing from the muffin tin.
7. Serve warm or store in an airtight container in the refrigerator for up to 3 days.

Nutritional Information (per muffin):

Total Carbohydrates: 1g | **Fiber:** 0g | **Sugars:** 0g | **Protein:** 8g | **Total Fat:** 2g | **Saturated Fat:** 1g | **Calories:** 50 | **Sodium:** 210mg | **Calcium:** 40mg | **Iron:** 0.3mg | **Vitamin B12:** 0.2mcg

Overnight Chia Pudding with Kiwi and Mango

Preparation Time: 10 minutes | Cooking Time: 0 minutes | Portion Size: 2 servings | Difficulty Level: Easy

Ingredients:

- ½ cup chia seeds
- 2 cups unsweetened almond milk
- 2 tablespoons honey
- 1 teaspoon vanilla extract
- 1 kiwi, peeled and diced
- ½ mango, peeled and diced
- Fresh mint leaves for garnish (optional)

Instructions:

1. In a bowl, combine chia seeds, almond milk, honey, and vanilla extract. Mix well.
2. Divide the mixture between two jars or bowls, cover, and refrigerate overnight or for at least 4 hours until the chia seeds have absorbed the liquid and the pudding is set.
3. Before serving, top each jar with diced kiwi and mango.
4. Garnish with fresh mint leaves if desired.
5. Serve chilled and enjoy!

Nutritional Information (per serving):

Total Carbohydrates: 32g | **Fiber:** 14g | **Sugars:** 15g | **Protein:** 7g | **Total Fat:** 9g | **Saturated**

Fat: 1g | **Calories:** 250 | **Sodium:** 150mg | **Calcium:** 250mg | **Iron:** 3mg | **Vitamin C:** 40mg

Berry and Greek Yogurt Smoothie

Preparation Time: 5 minutes | Cooking Time: 0 minutes | Portion Size: 2 servings | Difficulty Level: Easy

Ingredients:

- 1 cup frozen mixed berries
- ½ cup low-fat Greek yogurt
- 1 cup unsweetened almond milk
- 1 tablespoon honey
- 1 teaspoon vanilla extract
- 1 tablespoon chia seeds

Instructions:

1. In a blender, combine frozen mixed berries, Greek yogurt, almond milk, honey, vanilla extract, and chia seeds.

2. Blend until smooth and creamy.

3. Pour into two glasses and serve immediately.

Nutritional Information (per serving):

Total Carbohydrates: 28g | **Fiber:** 5g | **Sugars:** 15g | **Protein:** 8g | **Total Fat:** 3g | **Saturated Fat:** 1g | **Calories:** 150 | **Sodium:** 80mg | **Calcium:** 150mg | **Iron:** 1mg | **Vitamin C:** 30mg

Quinoa Porridge with Honey and Almonds

Preparation Time: 5 minutes | Cooking Time: 15 minutes | Portion Size: 2 servings | Difficulty Level: Easy

Ingredients:

- 1 cup cooked quinoa
- 1 cup unsweetened almond milk
- 2 tablespoons honey
- 1 teaspoon vanilla extract
- ½ teaspoon cinnamon
- 2 tablespoons sliced almonds
- Fresh berries for topping (optional)

Instructions:

1. In a medium saucepan, combine cooked quinoa, almond milk, honey, vanilla extract, and cinnamon.

2. Cook over medium heat, stirring occasionally, until the mixture begins to thicken, about 10-15 minutes.

3. Divide the quinoa porridge into two bowls.

4. Top with sliced almonds and fresh berries if desired.

5. Serve warm and enjoy!

Nutritional Information (per serving):

Total Carbohydrates: 40g | **Fiber:** 5g | **Sugars:** 15g | **Protein:** 7g | **Total Fat:** 7g | **Saturated Fat:** 1g | **Calories:** 230 | **Sodium:** 100mg | **Calcium:** 120mg | **Iron:** 2mg | **Vitamin B12:** 0.1mcg

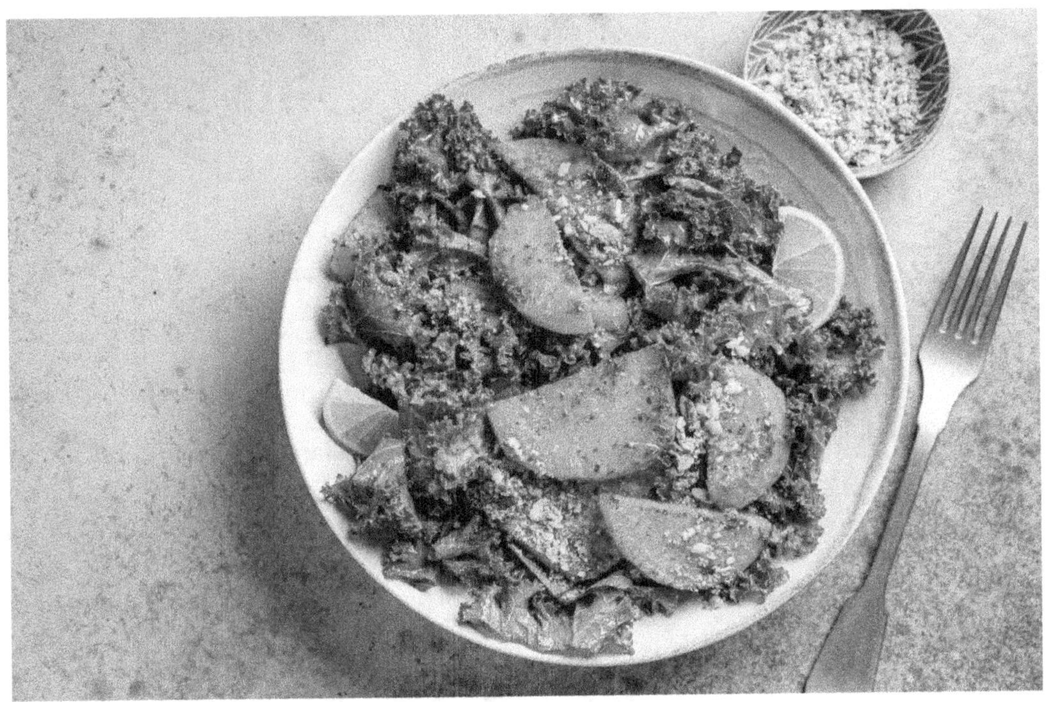

Baked Sweet Potato and Kale Hash

Preparation Time: 10 minutes | Cooking Time: 25 minutes | Portion Size: 4 servings | Difficulty Level: Easy

Ingredients:

- 2 medium sweet potatoes, peeled and diced
- 2 cups kale, chopped
- 1 red bell pepper, diced
- 1 small onion, diced
- 2 tablespoons olive oil
- 1 teaspoon smoked paprika
- ½ teaspoon cumin
- ½ teaspoon salt
- ¼ teaspoon black pepper

Instructions:

1. Preheat the oven to 400°F (200°C).

2. In a large bowl, toss the sweet potatoes, kale, bell pepper, onion, olive oil, smoked paprika, cumin, salt, and black pepper until well combined.

3. Spread the mixture evenly on a baking sheet lined with parchment paper.

4. Bake for 20-25 minutes, stirring halfway through, until the sweet potatoes are tender and slightly crisp.

5. Serve warm and enjoy!

Nutritional Information (per serving):

Total Carbohydrates: 25g | **Fiber:** 6g | **Sugars:** 7g | **Protein:** 2g | **Total Fat:** 7g | **Saturated Fat:** 1g | **Calories:** 170 | **Sodium:** 180mg | **Calcium:** 90mg | **Iron:** 1.5mg | **Vitamin C:** 40mg

Cottage Cheese and Pineapple Bowl

Preparation Time: 5 minutes | Cooking Time: 0 minutes | Portion Size: 2 bowls | Difficulty Level: Easy

Ingredients:

- 1 cup low-fat cottage cheese
- 1 cup fresh pineapple, diced
- 2 tablespoons shredded coconut
- 2 tablespoons chopped walnuts
- 1 tablespoon honey
- 1 teaspoon cinnamon

Instructions:

1. Divide the cottage cheese evenly between two bowls.
2. Top each bowl with diced pineapple, shredded coconut, and chopped walnuts.
3. Drizzle with honey and sprinkle with cinnamon.
4. Serve immediately and enjoy!

Nutritional Information (per bowl):

Total Carbohydrates: 20g | **Fiber:** 3g | **Sugars:** 15g | **Protein:** 12g | **Total Fat:** 5g | **Saturated Fat:** 2g | **Calories:** 150 | **Sodium:** 200mg | **Calcium:** 100mg | **Iron:** 0.5mg | **Vitamin C:** 35mg | **Vitamin B12:** 0.4mcg

Multigrain French Toast with Agave Syrup

Preparation Time: 10 minutes | Cooking Time: 15 minutes | Portion Size: 4 slices | Difficulty Level: Easy

Ingredients:

- 4 slices multigrain bread
- 2 large eggs
- ½ cup low-fat milk
- 1 teaspoon vanilla extract
- 1 teaspoon cinnamon
- Non-stick cooking spray
- 2 tablespoons agave syrup
- Fresh berries for topping

Instructions:

1. In a shallow bowl, whisk together eggs, low-fat milk, vanilla extract, and cinnamon.
2. Preheat a non-stick skillet over medium heat and spray with non-stick cooking spray.
3. Dip each slice of multigrain bread into the egg mixture, coating both sides.
4. Place the coated bread slices onto the skillet and cook until golden brown, about 2-3 minutes per side.
5. Remove from the skillet and repeat with the remaining slices.
6. Drizzle with agave syrup and top with fresh berries.
7. Serve immediately and enjoy!

Nutritional Information (per slice):

Total Carbohydrates: 30g | **Fiber:** 4g | **Sugars:** 10g | **Protein:** 8g | **Total Fat:** 5g | **Saturated Fat:** 1g | **Calories:** 200 | **Sodium:** 160mg | **Calcium:** 80mg | **Iron:** 2mg | **Vitamin B12:** 0.4mcg

Low-Fat Cottage Cheese Pancakes

Preparation Time: 10 minutes | Cooking Time: 15 minutes | Portion Size: 6 pancakes | Difficulty Level: Easy

Ingredients:

- 1 cup low-fat cottage cheese
- ½ cup whole wheat flour
- ½ cup rolled oats
- 2 large eggs
- 1 teaspoon baking powder
- 1 teaspoon vanilla extract
- 1 tablespoon honey
- ¼ teaspoon salt
- Non-stick cooking spray

Instructions:

1. In a blender, combine cottage cheese, whole wheat flour, rolled oats, eggs, baking powder, vanilla extract, honey, and salt. Blend until smooth.
2. Heat a non-stick skillet or griddle over medium heat and spray with non-stick cooking spray.
3. Pour ¼ cup of batter onto the skillet for each pancake. Cook until bubbles form on the surface and edges appear set, about 2-3 minutes. Flip and cook for another 1-2 minutes until golden brown.
4. Remove from the skillet and repeat with the remaining batter.
5. Serve warm with your favorite toppings.

Nutritional Information (per pancake):

Total Carbohydrates: 15g | **Fiber:** 2g | **Sugars:** 4g | **Protein:** 7g | **Total Fat:** 2g | **Saturated Fat:** 0.5g | **Calories:** 100 | **Sodium:** 160mg | **Calcium:** 60mg | **Iron:** 1mg | **Vitamin B12:** 0.2mcg

Smoked Salmon and Cream Cheese on a Bagel Thin

Preparation Time: 5 minutes | Cooking Time: 0 minutes | Portion Size: 2 bagel halves | Difficulty Level: Easy

Ingredients:

- 1 whole wheat bagel thin, split in half
- 2 tablespoons low-fat cream cheese
- 2 ounces smoked salmon
- 1 tablespoon capers
- ¼ cup arugula
- 1 teaspoon lemon juice
- Fresh dill for garnish
- Black pepper to taste

Instructions:

1. Spread low-fat cream cheese evenly over both halves of the bagel thin.
2. Layer smoked salmon on top of the cream cheese.
3. Sprinkle with capers and arugula.
4. Drizzle with lemon juice and garnish with fresh dill.
5. Season with black pepper to taste.
6. Serve immediately and enjoy!

Nutritional Information (per bagel half):

Total Carbohydrates: 23g | **Fiber:** 4g | **Sugars:** 2g | **Protein:** 10g | **Total Fat:** 5g | **Saturated Fat:** 1.5g | **Calories:** 150 | **Sodium:** 320mg | **Calcium:** 60mg | **Iron:** 1.2mg | **Vitamin B12:** 1.5mcg

Apple and Walnut Yogurt Parfait

Preparation Time: 10 minutes | Cooking Time: 0 minutes | Portion Size: 1 parfait | Difficulty Level: Easy

Ingredients:

- 1 cup low-fat Greek yogurt
- 1 apple, peeled and diced
- 2 tablespoons honey
- ¼ cup granola (low-fat, low-sugar)
- 2 tablespoons chopped walnuts
- 1 teaspoon cinnamon
- 1 teaspoon vanilla extract

Instructions:

1. In a small bowl, mix the Greek yogurt with honey, cinnamon, and vanilla extract until well combined.
2. In a parfait glass or a small bowl, layer ⅓ of the yogurt mixture at the bottom.
3. Add a layer of diced apple, granola, and chopped walnuts.
4. Repeat the layering process twice more, finishing with a layer of granola and a sprinkle of walnuts on top.
5. Serve immediately and enjoy!

Nutritional Information (per serving):

Total Carbohydrates: 35g | **Fiber:** 4g | **Sugars:** 18g | **Protein:** 12g | **Total Fat:** 8g | **Saturated Fat:** 1g | **Calories:** 240 | **Sodium:** 100mg | **Calcium:** 200mg | **Iron:** 1mg | **Vitamin B12:** 0.4mcg

Carrot and Hummus Roll-Ups

Preparation Time: 10 minutes | Cooking Time: 0 minutes | Portion Size: 4 roll-ups | Difficulty Level: Easy

Ingredients:

- 4 large whole wheat tortillas
- 1 cup hummus
- 2 large carrots, peeled and julienned
- 1 cucumber, julienned
- 1 red bell pepper, julienned
- 1 cup baby spinach leaves
- 1 teaspoon lemon juice
- Salt and pepper to taste

Instructions:

1. Lay the whole wheat tortillas flat on a clean surface.
2. Spread ¼ cup of hummus evenly on each tortilla.
3. Top each tortilla with julienned carrots, cucumber, bell pepper, and baby spinach leaves.
4. Drizzle with lemon juice and season with salt and pepper.
5. Roll up each tortilla tightly and slice into bite-sized pieces.
6. Serve immediately and enjoy!

Nutritional Information (per roll-up):

Total Carbohydrates: 22g | **Fiber:** 6g | **Sugars:** 3g | **Protein:** 6g | **Total Fat:** 5g | **Saturated Fat:** 1g | **Calories:** 150 | **Sodium:** 240mg | **Calcium:** 40mg | **Iron:** 1.5mg | **Vitamin C:** 15mg

Cucumber and Turkey Mini Sandwiches

Preparation Time: 10 minutes | Cooking Time: 0 minutes | Portion Size: 6 mini sandwiches | Difficulty Level: Easy

Ingredients:

- 1 cucumber, sliced into 12 thick rounds
- 6 slices deli turkey breast (low-sodium, nitrate-free), halved
- ¼ cup low-fat Greek yogurt
- 2 tablespoons mustard
- 1 tablespoon dill, finely chopped
- 1 teaspoon lemon juice
- Salt and pepper to taste
- Toothpicks for assembly

Instructions:

1. In a small bowl, mix the Greek yogurt, mustard, dill, lemon juice, salt, and pepper until well combined.
2. Spread the yogurt mixture onto one side of each cucumber round.
3. Fold each half-slice of turkey breast and place on top of 6 cucumber rounds.
4. Top with the remaining cucumber slices to form mini sandwiches.
5. Secure each mini sandwich with a toothpick.
6. Serve immediately or refrigerate for up to 2 hours before serving.

Nutritional Information (per mini sandwich):

Total Carbohydrates: 2g | **Fiber:** 0.5g | **Sugars:** 1g | **Protein:** 6g | **Total Fat:** 1g | **Saturated Fat:** 0.5g | **Calories:** 35 | **Sodium:** 150mg | **Calcium:** 10mg | **Iron:** 0.2mg

Greek Yogurt and Berry Compote

Preparation Time: 5 minutes | Cooking Time: 10 minutes | Portion Size: 2 servings | Difficulty Level: Easy

Ingredients:

- 2 cups low-fat Greek yogurt
- 1 cup mixed berries (fresh or frozen)
- 2 tablespoons honey
- 1 teaspoon lemon juice
- 1 teaspoon vanilla extract
- 1 teaspoon chia seeds (optional)
- Fresh mint leaves for garnish

Instructions:

1. In a small saucepan, combine mixed berries, honey, and lemon juice. Cook over medium heat, stirring occasionally, until the berries break down and the mixture thickens, about 8-10 minutes.

2. Remove from heat, stir in the vanilla extract, and let cool slightly.

3. Divide the Greek yogurt evenly between two bowls.

4. Top each bowl with the berry compote and sprinkle with chia seeds if desired.

5. Garnish with fresh mint leaves.

6. Serve immediately and enjoy!

Nutritional Information (per serving):

Total Carbohydrates: 25g | **Fiber:** 5g | **Sugars:** 18g | **Protein:** 12g | **Total Fat:** 3g | **Saturated Fat:** 1g | **Calories:** 180 | **Sodium:** 60mg | **Calcium:** 180mg | **Iron:** 1mg | **Vitamin C:** 25mg

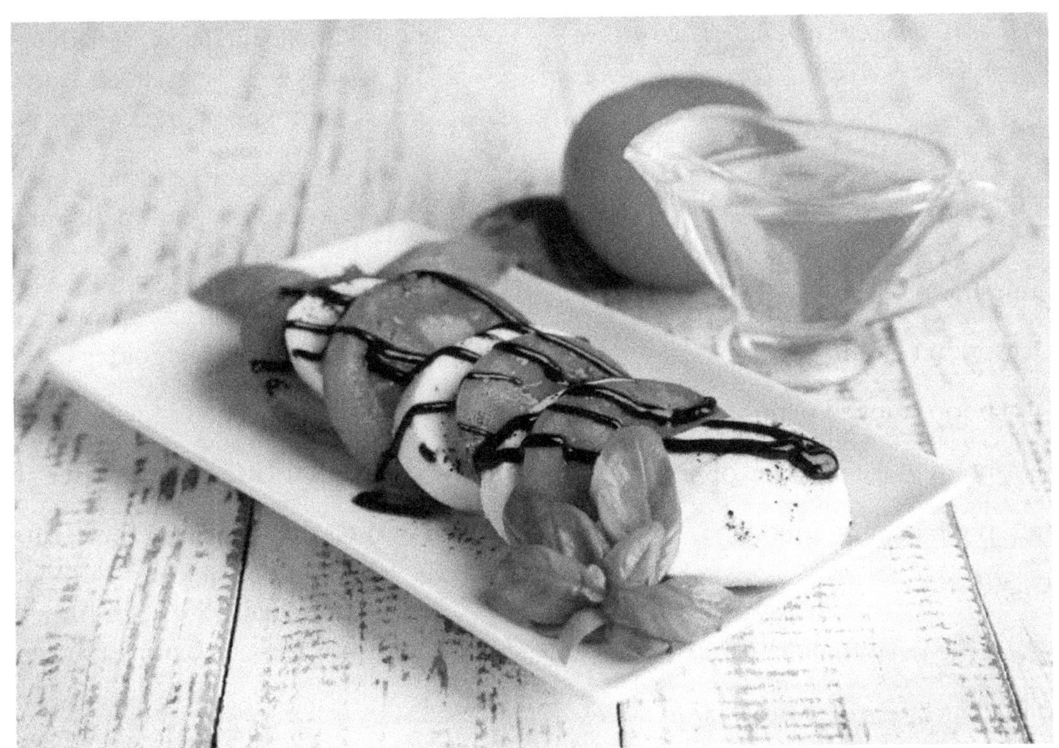

Caprese Salad Skewers with Balsamic Glaze

Preparation Time: 10 minutes | Cooking Time: 0 minutes | Portion Size: 12 skewers | Difficulty Level: Easy

Ingredients:

- 12 cherry tomatoes
- 12 small mozzarella balls (bocconcini)
- 12 fresh basil leaves
- 2 tablespoons balsamic glaze
- 1 tablespoon olive oil
- Salt and pepper to taste
- Toothpicks or small skewers

Instructions:

1. Thread one cherry tomato, one mozzarella ball, and one fresh basil leaf onto each toothpick or skewer.
2. Arrange the skewers on a serving plate.
3. Drizzle with olive oil and balsamic glaze.
4. Season with salt and pepper to taste.
5. Serve immediately and enjoy!

Nutritional Information (per skewer):

Total Carbohydrates: 3g | **Fiber:** 0.5g | **Sugars:** 2g | **Protein:** 4g | **Total Fat:** 5g | **Saturated Fat:** 2.5g | **Calories:** 70 | **Sodium:** 50mg | **Calcium:** 50mg | **Iron:** 0.2mg | **Vitamin C:** 4mg

Roasted Chickpeas with Sea Salt

Preparation Time: 10 minutes | Cooking Time: 40 minutes | Portion Size: 4 servings | Difficulty Level: Easy

Ingredients:

- 1 can (15 ounces) chickpeas, drained and rinsed
- 1 tablespoon olive oil
- ½ teaspoon sea salt
- ½ teaspoon smoked paprika (optional)
- ¼ teaspoon garlic powder (optional)
- ¼ teaspoon cumin (optional)

Instructions:

1. Preheat the oven to 400°F (200°C).
2. Pat the chickpeas dry with a clean towel. The drier they are, the crispier they will be.
3. In a large bowl, toss the chickpeas with olive oil, sea salt, and any desired spices (smoked paprika, garlic powder, cumin).
4. Spread the chickpeas evenly on a baking sheet lined with parchment paper.
5. Roast in the oven for 35-40 minutes, stirring halfway through, until the chickpeas are golden and crispy.
6. Let cool for a few minutes before serving.

Nutritional Information (per serving):

Total Carbohydrates: 16g | **Fiber:** 5g | **Sugars:** 1g | **Protein:** 5g | **Total Fat:** 5g | **Saturated Fat:** 0.5g | **Calories:** 120 | **Sodium:** 200mg | **Calcium:** 30mg | **Iron:** 1.5mg

Avocado and Shrimp Salad Cups

Preparation Time: 15 minutes | Cooking Time: 5 minutes | Portion Size: 6 cups | Difficulty Level: Easy

Ingredients:

- 1 large avocado, diced
- 12 cooked shrimp, peeled and deveined
- ½ cup cherry tomatoes, halved
- ½ cucumber, diced
- 2 tablespoons red onion, finely chopped
- 2 tablespoons cilantro, chopped
- 2 tablespoons lime juice
- 1 tablespoon olive oil
- Salt and pepper to taste
- 6 large lettuce leaves

Instructions:

1. In a large bowl, combine the avocado, shrimp, cherry tomatoes, cucumber, red onion, cilantro, lime juice, and olive oil.
2. Season with salt and pepper to taste.
3. Toss gently until all ingredients are well coated.
4. Place one lettuce leaf on each serving plate and fill with the avocado and shrimp salad mixture.
5. Serve immediately and enjoy!

Nutritional Information (per cup):

Total Carbohydrates: 5g | **Fiber:** 2g | **Sugars:** 1g | **Protein:** 10g | **Total Fat:** 7g | **Saturated Fat:** 1g | **Calories:** 110 | **Sodium:** 200mg | **Calcium:** 40mg | **Iron:** 1mg

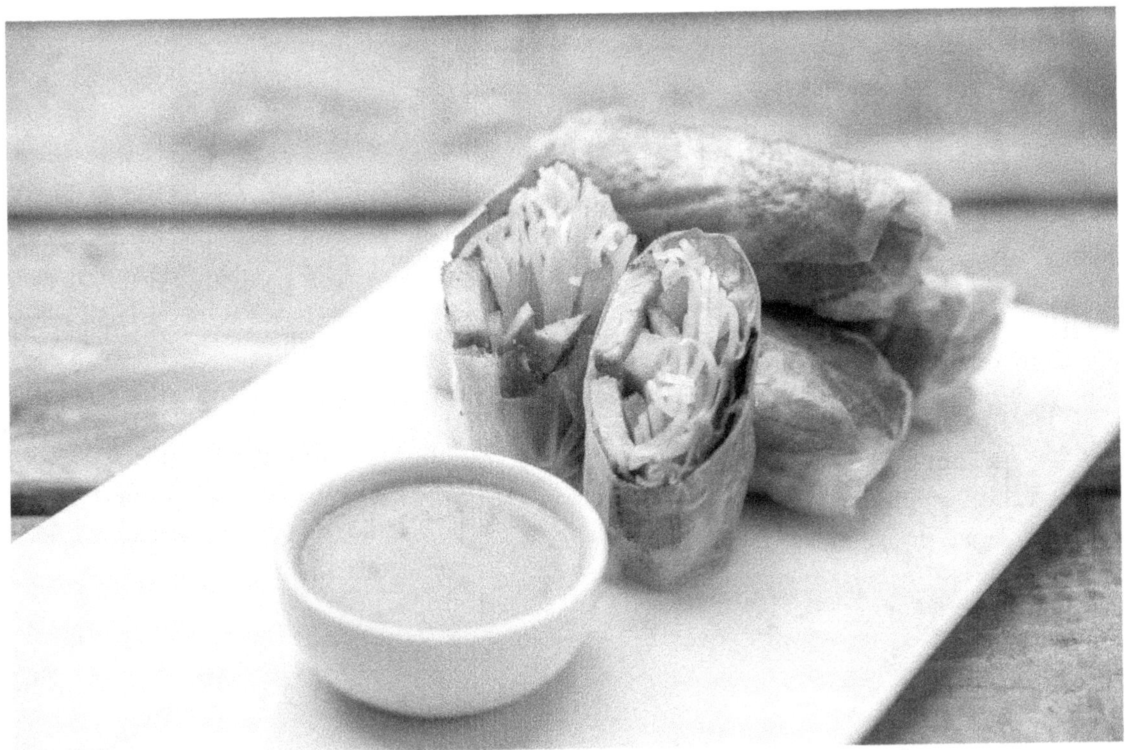

Vegetable Spring Rolls with Peanut Dipping Sauce

Preparation Time: 20 minutes | Cooking Time: 0 minutes | Portion Size: 8 rolls | Difficulty Level: Medium

Ingredients:

Spring Rolls:

- 8 rice paper wrappers
- 1 cup vermicelli rice noodles, cooked and drained
- 1 carrot, julienned
- 1 cucumber, julienned
- 1 bell pepper, julienned
- 1 avocado, sliced
- 1 cup fresh mint leaves
- 1 cup fresh cilantro leaves
- 1 cup fresh basil leaves

Peanut Dipping Sauce:

- ¼ cup peanut butter
- 2 tablespoons soy sauce (low-sodium)
- 2 tablespoons lime juice
- 1 tablespoon honey
- 1 teaspoon sesame oil
- 1 teaspoon sriracha sauce (optional)
- Warm water as needed for thinning

Instructions:

1. **Prepare the Spring Rolls:**

   1. Fill a shallow dish with warm water. Dip one rice paper wrapper into the water for about 10 seconds or until pliable.

   2. Lay the softened wrapper on a clean surface and arrange a small amount of vermicelli noodles, carrot, cucumber, bell pepper, avocado, mint leaves, cilantro

leaves, and basil leaves in the center.

3. Fold the bottom of the wrapper over the filling, then fold in the sides and roll tightly to seal.

4. Repeat with the remaining wrappers and filling ingredients.

2. **Make the Peanut Dipping Sauce:**

   1. In a small bowl, whisk together peanut butter, soy sauce, lime juice, honey, sesame oil, and sriracha sauce (if using).

   2. Add warm water a little at a time to achieve desired consistency.

3. **Serve:**

   1. Arrange the spring rolls on a serving plate and serve with the peanut dipping sauce.

   2. Enjoy immediately.

Nutritional Information (per roll with sauce):

Total Carbohydrates: 18g | **Fiber:** 3g | **Sugars:** 5g | **Protein:** 4g | **Total Fat:** 6g | **Saturated Fat:** 1g | **Calories:** 140 | **Sodium:** 250mg | **Calcium:** 30mg | **Iron:** 1mg

Spiced Pumpkin Seeds

Preparation Time: 5 minutes | Cooking Time: 20 minutes | Portion Size: 4 servings | Difficulty Level: Easy

Ingredients:

- 1 cup raw pumpkin seeds
- 1 tablespoon olive oil
- ½ teaspoon smoked paprika
- ½ teaspoon garlic powder
- ½ teaspoon cumin
- ¼ teaspoon cayenne pepper (optional)
- ¼ teaspoon sea salt

Instructions:

1. Preheat the oven to 350°F (180°C).

2. In a bowl, toss the pumpkin seeds with olive oil, smoked paprika, garlic powder, cumin, cayenne pepper (if using), and sea salt until well coated.

3. Spread the pumpkin seeds evenly on a baking sheet lined with parchment paper.

4. Bake in the oven for 15-20 minutes, stirring halfway through, until golden and crispy.

5. Let cool for a few minutes before serving.

Nutritional Information (per serving):

Total Carbohydrates: 4g | **Fiber:** 2g | **Sugars:** 0g | **Protein:** 5g | **Total Fat:** 10g | **Saturated Fat:** 1.5g | **Calories:** 130 | **Sodium:** 100mg | **Calcium:** 10mg | **Iron:** 1mg | **Vitamin C:** 0mg

Baked Apple Chips

Preparation Time: 10 minutes | Cooking Time: 2 hours | Portion Size: 4 servings | Difficulty Level: Easy

Ingredients:

- 2 large apples (Gala or Honeycrisp)

- 1 teaspoon cinnamon

- 1 teaspoon sugar (optional)

Instructions:

1. Preheat the oven to 200°F (95°C).

2. Line two baking sheets with parchment paper.

3. Wash and core the apples, then slice them thinly (about ⅛ inch) using a mandoline or sharp knife.

4. Arrange the apple slices in a single layer on the baking sheets.

5. In a small bowl, mix cinnamon and sugar (if using) together. Sprinkle evenly over the apple slices.

6. Bake for 1 hour, then flip the apple slices and bake for another hour until the apples are dry and crispy.

7. Turn off the oven and leave the apple chips inside for 1 hour to crisp up further.

8. Let cool completely before serving or storing in an airtight container.

Nutritional Information (per serving):

Total Carbohydrates: 20g | **Fiber:** 3g | **Sugars:** 15g | **Protein:** 0g | **Total Fat:** 0g | **Saturated Fat:** 0g | **Calories:** 80 | **Sodium:** 0mg | **Calcium:** 10mg | **Iron:** 0.3mg

Sweet Potato and Black Bean Quesadillas

Preparation Time: 15 minutes | Cooking Time: 15 minutes | Portion Size: 4 quesadillas | Difficulty Level: Easy

Ingredients:

- 2 medium sweet potatoes, peeled and diced

- 1 cup black beans, cooked and drained

- 1 cup low-fat shredded cheddar cheese

- 1 teaspoon cumin

- ½ teaspoon chili powder

- ½ teaspoon smoked paprika

- ¼ teaspoon salt

- ¼ teaspoon black pepper

- 8 whole wheat tortillas

- 2 tablespoons olive oil

- Fresh cilantro, chopped (for garnish)

- Lime wedges (for serving)

Instructions:

1. In a large pot, bring salted water to a boil and add diced sweet potatoes. Cook for about 10 minutes until tender. Drain and transfer to a bowl.

2. Mash the sweet potatoes with a fork, then stir in black beans, cumin, chili powder, smoked paprika, salt, and black pepper.

3. Place a tortilla on a flat surface and spread a quarter of the sweet potato mixture evenly over one half of the tortilla. Sprinkle with ¼ cup shredded cheddar cheese, then fold the tortilla in half. Repeat with the remaining tortillas.

4. Heat 1 tablespoon of olive oil in a non-stick skillet over medium heat. Add two folded tortillas to the skillet and cook for 2-3 minutes on each side until golden brown and the cheese is melted.

5. Remove the quesadillas from the skillet and repeat with the remaining olive oil and tortillas.

6. Cut each quesadilla into wedges and garnish with chopped cilantro.

7. Serve with lime wedges and enjoy!

Nutritional Information (per quesadilla):

Total Carbohydrates: 40g | **Fiber:** 8g | **Sugars:** 6g | **Protein:** 14g | **Total Fat:** 12g | **Saturated Fat:** 4g | **Calories:** 290 | **Sodium:** 450mg | **Calcium:** 180mg | **Iron:** 2.5mg

Tuna Salad Stuffed Tomatoes

Preparation Time: 10 minutes | Cooking Time: 0 minutes | Portion Size: 4 servings | Difficulty Level: Easy

Ingredients:

- 4 large tomatoes
- 2 cans (5 ounces each) tuna in water, drained
- ¼ cup low-fat Greek yogurt
- 2 tablespoons low-fat mayonnaise
- 2 tablespoons red onion, finely chopped
- 2 tablespoons celery, finely chopped
- 1 tablespoon parsley, finely chopped
- 1 teaspoon Dijon mustard
- 1 teaspoon lemon juice
- Salt and pepper to taste

Instructions:

1. Slice the tops off the tomatoes and scoop out the pulp and seeds, creating hollow cavities. Set aside.

2. In a medium bowl, combine drained tuna, Greek yogurt, mayonnaise, red onion, celery, parsley, Dijon mustard, lemon juice, salt, and pepper. Mix until well combined.

3. Fill each hollowed tomato with the tuna salad mixture.

4. Serve immediately or refrigerate for up to 2 hours before serving.

Nutritional Information (per serving):

Total Carbohydrates: 6g | **Fiber:** 2g | **Sugars:** 4g | **Protein:** 18g | **Total Fat:** 4g | **Saturated Fat:** 1g | **Calories:** 130 | **Sodium:** 260mg | **Calcium:** 40mg | **Iron:** 1mg | **Vitamin C:** 15mg

Chicken Lettuce Wraps with Mango Salsa

Preparation Time: 15 minutes | Cooking Time: 10 minutes | Portion Size: 4 servings | Difficulty Level: Easy

Ingredients:

Chicken Lettuce Wraps:

- 1 pound ground chicken
- 1 tablespoon olive oil
- 2 cloves garlic, minced
- 1 tablespoon soy sauce (low-sodium)
- 1 tablespoon hoisin sauce
- 1 teaspoon sesame oil
- ½ teaspoon ginger, grated
- Salt and pepper to taste

- 8 large lettuce leaves (e.g., butter, romaine)

Mango Salsa:

- 1 ripe mango, diced
- ½ red bell pepper, diced
- ¼ cup red onion, finely chopped
- ¼ cup cilantro, chopped
- 1 tablespoon lime juice
- 1 teaspoon olive oil
- Salt and pepper to taste

Instructions:

1. **Prepare the Mango Salsa:**

   1. In a medium bowl, combine mango, red bell pepper, red onion, cilantro, lime juice, olive oil, salt, and pepper.
   2. Mix well and set aside.

2. **Cook the Chicken Filling:**

   1. In a large skillet, heat olive oil over medium heat. Add minced garlic and sauté for 1 minute until fragrant.
   2. Add ground chicken and cook until no longer pink, about 5-7 minutes.
   3. Stir in soy sauce, hoisin sauce, sesame oil, grated ginger, salt, and pepper. Cook for another 2 minutes.
   4. Remove from heat.

3. **Assemble the Lettuce Wraps:**

   1. Place a spoonful of the chicken mixture into each lettuce leaf.
   2. Top with mango salsa.
   3. Serve immediately and enjoy!

Nutritional Information (per serving):

Total Carbohydrates: 14g | **Fiber:** 3g | **Sugars:** 9g | **Protein:** 20g | **Total Fat:** 8g | **Saturated Fat:** 2g | **Calories:** 180 | **Sodium:** 340mg | **Calcium:** 30mg | **Iron:** 1.5mg

Broccoli and Cheese Mini Quiches

Preparation Time: 15 minutes | Cooking Time: 20 minutes | Portion Size: 12 mini quiches | Difficulty Level: Medium

Ingredients:

- 1 cup broccoli florets, finely chopped
- 1 cup low-fat shredded cheddar cheese
- 4 large eggs
- 1 cup low-fat milk
- ¼ teaspoon garlic powder
- ¼ teaspoon onion powder
- ¼ teaspoon salt
- ¼ teaspoon black pepper
- Non-stick cooking spray

Instructions:

1. Preheat the oven to 350°F (180°C). Spray a muffin tin with non-stick cooking spray.
2. In a large bowl, whisk together eggs, low-fat milk, garlic powder, onion powder, salt, and black pepper.
3. Divide the chopped broccoli florets evenly among the 12 muffin cups.
4. Sprinkle shredded cheddar cheese on top of the broccoli in each cup.

5. Pour the egg mixture over the broccoli and cheese, filling each muffin cup about three-quarters full.

6. Bake for 18-20 minutes or until the mini quiches are set and lightly browned.

7. Let cool slightly before removing from the muffin tin.

8. Serve warm or store in an airtight container in the refrigerator for up to 3 days.

Nutritional Information (per mini quiche):

Total Carbohydrates: 2g | **Fiber:** 0.5g | **Sugars:** 1g | **Protein:** 5g | **Total Fat:** 4g | **Saturated Fat:** 1.5g | **Calories:** 60 | **Sodium:** 120mg | **Calcium:** 70mg | **Iron:** 0.3mg | **Vitamin C:** 10mg

Mozzarella and Tomato Basil Bruschetta

Preparation Time: 10 minutes | Cooking Time: 5 minutes | Portion Size: 8 pieces | Difficulty Level: Easy

Ingredients:

- 8 slices whole wheat baguette

- 1 clove garlic, halved

- 2 tablespoons olive oil

- 1 cup cherry tomatoes, diced

- ½ cup low-fat mozzarella cheese, diced

- ¼ cup fresh basil leaves, chopped

- 1 tablespoon balsamic vinegar

- Salt and pepper to taste

Instructions:

1. Preheat the oven to 400°F (200°C).

2. Arrange the baguette slices on a baking sheet. Rub each slice with the cut side of the garlic clove and brush lightly with olive oil.

3. Toast the baguette slices in the oven for 5 minutes or until golden and crisp.

4. In a medium bowl, combine cherry tomatoes, mozzarella cheese, basil leaves, balsamic vinegar, salt, and pepper.

5. Spoon the tomato and mozzarella mixture evenly over the toasted baguette slices.

6. Serve immediately and enjoy!

Nutritional Information (per piece):

Total Carbohydrates: 10g | **Fiber:** 1g | **Sugars:** 1g | **Protein:** 4g | **Total Fat:** 3g | **Saturated Fat:** 1g | **Calories:** 90 | **Sodium:** 120mg | **Calcium:** 40mg | **Iron:** 0.5mg

Hard-Boiled Egg and Avocado Bowl

Preparation Time: 10 minutes | Cooking Time: 10 minutes | Portion Size: 2 bowls | Difficulty Level: Easy

Ingredients:

- 4 large eggs

- 1 large avocado, diced

- 1 cup cherry tomatoes, halved

- 2 cups mixed greens

- 1 tablespoon lemon juice

- 1 tablespoon olive oil

- Salt and pepper to taste

- Fresh parsley, chopped (for garnish)

Instructions:

1. Place the eggs in a saucepan and cover with water. Bring to a boil over medium-high heat. Once boiling, cover, remove from heat, and let sit for 10 minutes.

2. Drain the eggs and transfer them to a bowl of ice water to cool. Once cooled, peel and slice the eggs.

3. In a medium bowl, combine avocado, cherry tomatoes, mixed greens, lemon juice, olive oil, salt, and pepper. Toss gently to combine.

4. Divide the salad mixture evenly between two bowls.

5. Top each bowl with sliced eggs and garnish with chopped parsley.

6. Serve immediately and enjoy!

Nutritional Information (per bowl):

Total Carbohydrates: 10g | **Fiber:** 4g | **Sugars:** 3g | **Protein:** 10g | **Total Fat:** 14g | **Saturated Fat:** 3g | **Calories:** 200 | **Sodium:** 120mg | **Calcium:** 50mg | **Iron:** 2mg

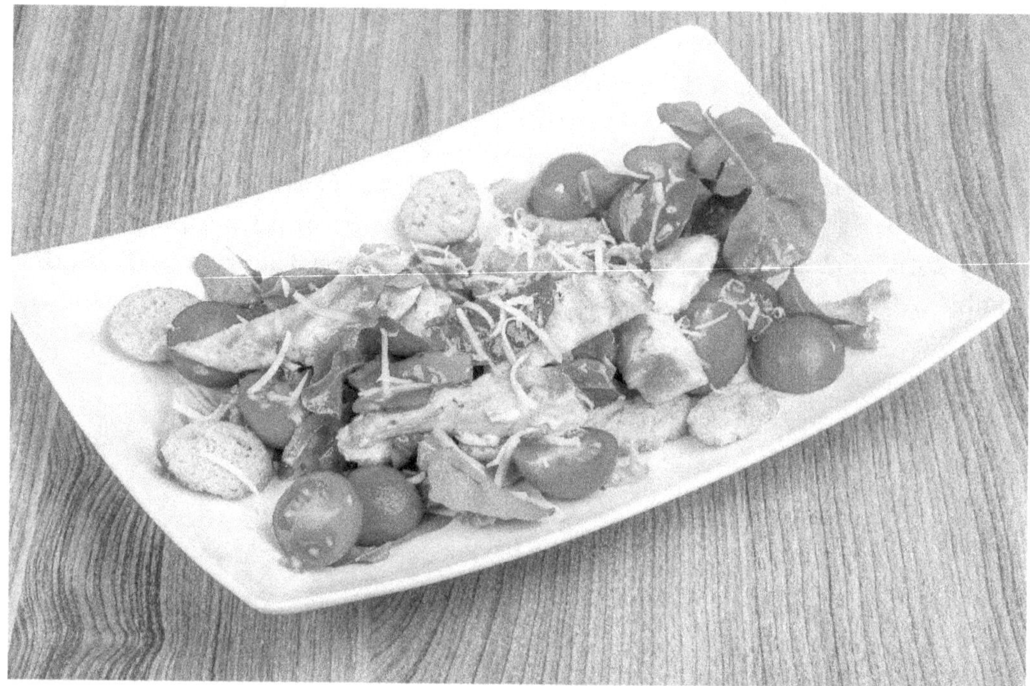

Grilled Chicken Caesar Salad with Low-Fat Dressing

Preparation Time: 15 minutes | Cooking Time: 10 minutes | Portion Size: 2 servings | Difficulty Level: Easy

Ingredients:

Salad:

- 2 boneless, skinless chicken breasts
- 4 cups romaine lettuce, chopped
- ½ cup cherry tomatoes, halved
- ¼ cup croutons (whole wheat)
- 2 tablespoons Parmesan cheese, grated
- Salt and pepper to taste
- Olive oil spray

Low-Fat Dressing:

- ¼ cup low-fat Greek yogurt
- 1 tablespoon lemon juice
- 1 tablespoon Dijon mustard
- 1 clove garlic, minced
- 1 teaspoon Worcestershire sauce
- ½ teaspoon anchovy paste (optional)
- Salt and pepper to taste

Instructions:

1. **Prepare the Dressing:**

   1. In a small bowl, whisk together Greek yogurt, lemon juice, Dijon mustard, garlic, Worcestershire sauce, anchovy paste (if using), salt, and pepper.

   2. Set aside.

2. **Grill the Chicken:**

1. Preheat the grill to medium-high heat. Lightly spray the chicken breasts with olive oil and season with salt and pepper.

2. Grill the chicken breasts for 5-7 minutes on each side, or until fully cooked.

3. Remove from the grill and let rest for 5 minutes before slicing.

3. **Assemble the Salad:**

   1. In a large bowl, toss together romaine lettuce, cherry tomatoes, croutons, and Parmesan cheese.

   2. Divide the salad between two bowls.

   3. Top each bowl with grilled chicken slices.

   4. Drizzle with the low-fat dressing and serve immediately.

Nutritional Information (per serving):

Total Carbohydrates: 18g | **Fiber:** 4g | **Sugars:** 5g | **Protein:** 28g | **Total Fat:** 8g | **Saturated Fat:** 2g | **Calories:** 230 | **Sodium:** 320mg | **Calcium:** 100mg | **Iron:** 2.5mg

Quinoa Tabbouleh with Lemon and Herbs

Preparation Time: 15 minutes | Cooking Time: 15 minutes | Portion Size: 4 servings | Difficulty Level: Easy

Ingredients:

- 1 cup quinoa, rinsed
- 2 cups water
- 1 cup parsley, finely chopped
- ½ cup mint leaves, finely chopped
- 1 cucumber, diced
- 2 tomatoes, diced
- ¼ cup red onion, finely chopped
- ¼ cup lemon juice
- 2 tablespoons olive oil
- Salt and pepper to taste

Instructions:

1. **Cook the Quinoa:**

   1. In a medium saucepan, combine quinoa and water. Bring to a boil over medium-high heat.

   2. Reduce the heat to low, cover, and simmer for 15 minutes, or until the water is absorbed.

   3. Remove from heat, fluff with a fork, and let cool.

2. **Prepare the Tabbouleh:**

   1. In a large bowl, combine cooled quinoa, parsley, mint leaves, cucumber, tomatoes, and red onion.

   2. In a small bowl, whisk together lemon juice, olive oil, salt, and pepper.

   3. Pour the dressing over the quinoa mixture and toss gently to combine.

3. **Serve:**

   1. Divide the tabbouleh evenly among four plates.

2. Serve immediately or refrigerate for up to 2 days.

Nutritional Information (per serving):

Total Carbohydrates: 28g | **Fiber:** 4g | **Sugars:** 3g | **Protein:** 6g | **Total Fat:** 6g | **Saturated Fat:** 1g | **Calories:** 180 | **Sodium:** 100mg | **Calcium:** 40mg | **Iron:** 2mg

Turkey and Avocado Wrap with Whole Wheat Tortilla

Preparation Time: 10 minutes | Cooking Time: 0 minutes | Portion Size: 2 wraps | Difficulty Level: Easy

Ingredients:

- 2 whole wheat tortillas
- 6 slices deli turkey breast (low-sodium, nitrate-free)
- 1 large avocado, sliced
- ½ cup lettuce, shredded
- ¼ cup cherry tomatoes, halved
- ¼ cup cucumber, sliced
- 2 tablespoons hummus
- 1 tablespoon lemon juice
- Salt and pepper to taste

Instructions:

1. Lay the whole wheat tortillas flat on a clean surface.
2. Spread 1 tablespoon of hummus on each tortilla.
3. Layer 3 slices of turkey breast, avocado slices, shredded lettuce, cherry tomatoes, and cucumber on each tortilla.
4. Drizzle with lemon juice and season with salt and pepper.
5. Roll up each tortilla tightly and slice in half.
6. Serve immediately and enjoy!

Nutritional Information (per wrap):

Total Carbohydrates: 28g | **Fiber:** 7g | **Sugars:** 3g | **Protein:** 16g | **Total Fat:** 10g | **Saturated Fat:** 1.5g | **Calories:** 250 | **Sodium:** 350mg | **Calcium:** 40mg | **Iron:** 2mg

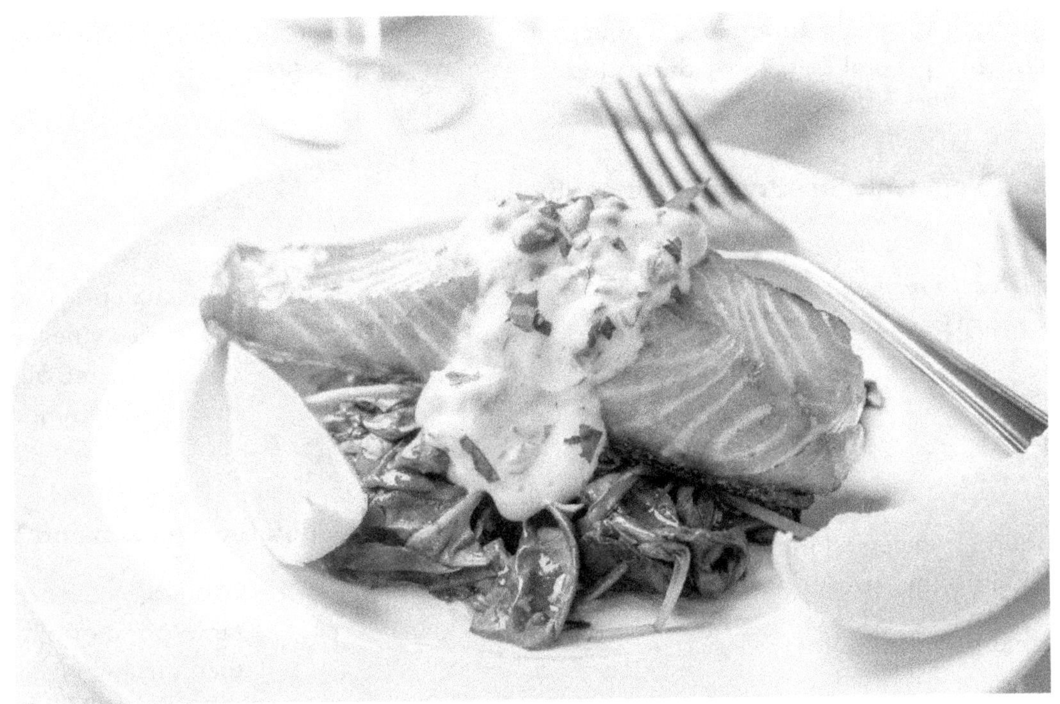

Baked Salmon with Dill and Lemon over Greens

Preparation Time: 10 minutes | Cooking Time: 15 minutes | Portion Size: 4 servings | Difficulty Level: Easy

Ingredients:

- 4 salmon fillets (6 ounces each)
- 2 tablespoons olive oil
- 1 lemon, thinly sliced
- 2 tablespoons fresh dill, chopped
- Salt and pepper to taste
- 4 cups mixed greens (such as arugula, spinach, and kale)
- 1 tablespoon lemon juice (for dressing)
- 1 teaspoon Dijon mustard (for dressing)
- 3 tablespoons extra virgin olive oil (for dressing)

Instructions:

1. Preheat the oven to 400°F (200°C).
2. Place the salmon fillets on a baking sheet lined with parchment paper.
3. Drizzle each fillet with olive oil and season with salt and pepper.
4. Top each fillet with a few lemon slices and sprinkle with chopped dill.
5. Bake in the preheated oven for 12-15 minutes, or until salmon is cooked through and flakes easily with a fork.
6. While the salmon is baking, prepare the salad dressing by whisking together lemon juice, Dijon mustard, and extra virgin olive oil in a small bowl.
7. Toss the mixed greens with the dressing in a large bowl.
8. Serve the baked salmon over the dressed greens.
9. Enjoy immediately!

Nutritional Information (per serving):

Total Carbohydrates: 5g | **Fiber:** 2g | **Sugars:** 1g | **Protein:** 24g | **Total Fat:** 15g | **Saturated** **Fat:** 2g | **Calories:** 290 | **Sodium:** 180mg | **Calcium:** 50mg | **Iron:** 1.5mg

Chicken and Vegetable Stir-Fry with Ginger Sauce

Preparation Time: 15 minutes | Cooking Time: 15 minutes | Portion Size: 4 servings | Difficulty Level: Medium

Ingredients:

Stir-Fry:

- 1 pound boneless, skinless chicken breast, sliced into thin strips
- 2 tablespoons olive oil
- 1 onion, sliced
- 1 red bell pepper, sliced
- 1 yellow bell pepper, sliced
- 1 zucchini, sliced
- 1 cup broccoli florets
- 1 cup snow peas
- 2 cloves garlic, minced
- 1 tablespoon sesame seeds (optional)

Ginger Sauce:

- ¼ cup low-sodium soy sauce
- 2 tablespoons rice vinegar
- 2 tablespoons honey
- 1 tablespoon fresh ginger, grated
- 1 teaspoon sesame oil
- 1 teaspoon cornstarch

Instructions:

1. **Prepare the Ginger Sauce:**

   1. In a small bowl, whisk together soy sauce, rice vinegar, honey, grated ginger, sesame oil, and cornstarch until well combined.
   2. Set aside.

2. **Cook the Chicken and Vegetables:**

   1. In a large skillet or wok, heat 1 tablespoon of olive oil over medium-high heat.
   2. Add sliced chicken and cook for 5-6 minutes until fully cooked and no longer pink. Remove chicken from the skillet and set aside.
   3. Add the remaining olive oil to the skillet. Add onion, red bell pepper, yellow bell pepper, zucchini, broccoli florets, snow peas, and garlic. Sauté for 5-6 minutes until the vegetables are tender-crisp.
   4. Return the cooked chicken to the skillet and pour in the ginger sauce. Stir well to combine.
   5. Cook for another 2-3 minutes until the sauce has thickened.

3. **Serve:**

   1. Garnish the stir-fry with sesame seeds (if using) and serve immediately.

Nutritional Information (per serving):

Total Carbohydrates: 15g | **Fiber:** 4g | **Sugars:** 8g | **Protein:** 28g | **Total Fat:** 9g | **Saturated Fat:** 1.5g | **Calories:** 250 | **Sodium:** 470mg | **Calcium:** 60mg | **Iron:** 2mg

Pasta Primavera with Olive Oil and Parmesan

Preparation Time: 15 minutes | Cooking Time: 15 minutes | Portion Size: 4 servings | Difficulty Level: Easy

Ingredients:

- 8 ounces whole wheat pasta (penne or spaghetti)
- 2 tablespoons olive oil
- 2 cloves garlic, minced
- 1 small zucchini, diced
- 1 small yellow squash, diced
- 1 cup cherry tomatoes, halved
- 1 red bell pepper, diced
- 1 cup broccoli florets
- ½ cup green peas (fresh or frozen)
- ¼ cup fresh basil leaves, chopped
- ¼ cup Parmesan cheese, grated
- Salt and pepper to taste

Instructions:

1. **Cook the Pasta:**

   1. In a large pot of salted boiling water, cook pasta according to package instructions until al dente. Drain and set aside.

2. **Prepare the Vegetables:**

   1. In a large skillet, heat olive oil over medium heat.

   2. Add garlic and sauté for 1 minute until fragrant.

   3. Add zucchini, yellow squash, cherry tomatoes, red bell pepper, broccoli florets, and green peas. Sauté for 5-6 minutes until the vegetables are tender-crisp.

3. **Combine and Serve:**

   1. Add the cooked pasta to the skillet and toss gently to combine.

   2. Season with salt and pepper to taste.

   3. Remove from heat and stir in chopped basil leaves.

   4. Divide the pasta among four plates and sprinkle with Parmesan cheese.

   5. Serve immediately and enjoy!

Nutritional Information (per serving):

Total Carbohydrates: 50g | **Fiber:** 8g | **Sugars:** 6g | **Protein:** 12g | **Total Fat:** 10g | **Saturated Fat:** 2.5g | **Calories:** 320 | **Sodium:** 150mg | **Calcium:** 100mg | **Iron:** 3mg

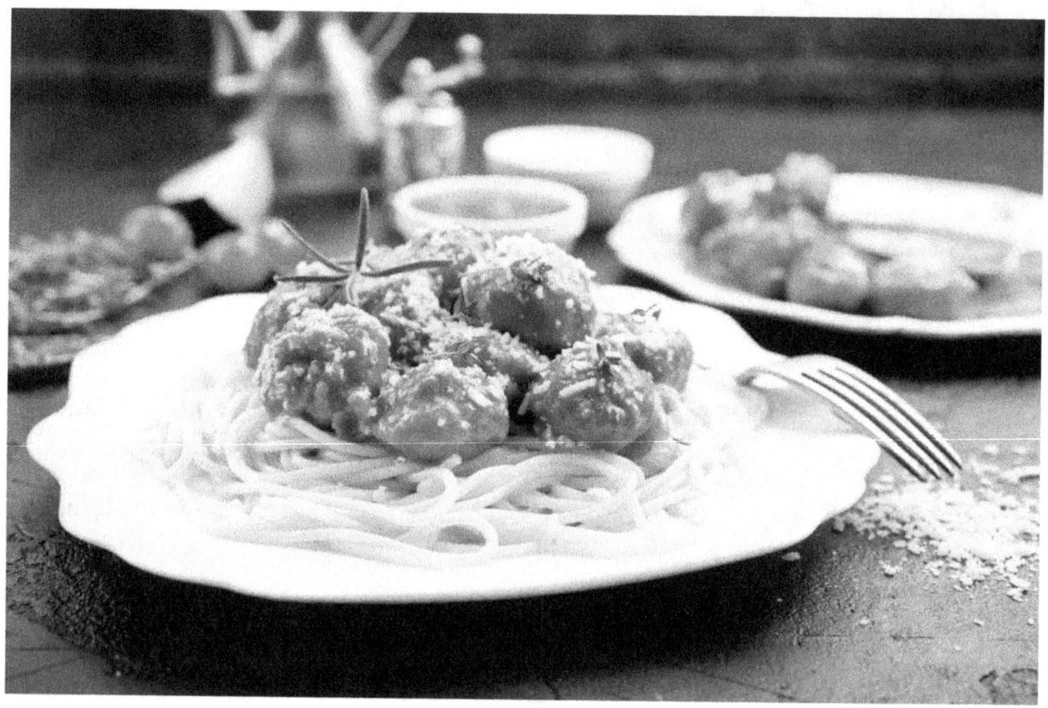

Turkey Meatballs in Marinara Sauce over Spaghetti Squash

Preparation Time: 15 minutes | Cooking Time: 45 minutes | Portion Size: 4 servings | Difficulty Level: Medium

Ingredients:

Spaghetti Squash:

- 1 medium spaghetti squash
- 1 tablespoon olive oil
- Salt and pepper to taste

Turkey Meatballs:

- 1 pound ground turkey
- 1 egg, beaten
- ½ cup whole wheat breadcrumbs
- 2 tablespoons Parmesan cheese, grated
- 1 teaspoon Italian seasoning
- ½ teaspoon garlic powder
- ½ teaspoon onion powder
- ½ teaspoon salt
- ¼ teaspoon black pepper

Marinara Sauce:

- 1 tablespoon olive oil
- 1 onion, diced
- 2 cloves garlic, minced
- 1 can (15 ounces) crushed tomatoes
- 1 teaspoon Italian seasoning
- ½ teaspoon salt
- ¼ teaspoon black pepper
- Fresh basil, chopped (for garnish)

Instructions:

1. **Prepare the Spaghetti Squash:**

    1. Preheat the oven to 400°F (200°C).

    2. Cut the spaghetti squash in half lengthwise and scoop out the seeds.

    3. Drizzle the cut sides with olive oil, and season with salt and pepper.

4. Place the squash halves cut side down on a baking sheet lined with parchment paper.

5. Roast for 35-40 minutes, or until the squash is tender.

6. Let cool slightly, then use a fork to scrape out the spaghetti-like strands.

2. **Prepare the Turkey Meatballs:**

   1. In a large bowl, combine ground turkey, beaten egg, breadcrumbs, Parmesan cheese, Italian seasoning, garlic powder, onion powder, salt, and black pepper.

   2. Mix well and form into 12-14 meatballs.

   3. Place the meatballs on a baking sheet lined with parchment paper.

   4. Bake in the preheated oven at 400°F (200°C) for 15-18 minutes until fully cooked.

3. **Prepare the Marinara Sauce:**

   1. In a large skillet, heat olive oil over medium heat. Add onion and garlic, and sauté for 3-4 minutes until softened.

   2. Stir in crushed tomatoes, Italian seasoning, salt, and black pepper.

   3. Bring to a simmer and cook for 10 minutes, stirring occasionally.

   4. Add the cooked turkey meatballs to the marinara sauce and simmer for another 5 minutes.

4. **Serve:**

   1. Divide the spaghetti squash strands evenly among four plates.

   2. Spoon the turkey meatballs and marinara sauce over the spaghetti squash.

   3. Garnish with fresh basil and serve immediately.

Nutritional Information (per serving):

Total Carbohydrates: 20g | **Fiber:** 4g | **Sugars:** 7g | **Protein:** 25g | **Total Fat:** 10g | **Saturated Fat:** 2g | **Calories:** 290 | **Sodium:** 450mg | **Calcium:** 80mg | **Iron:** 3mg

Roasted Beet and Goat Cheese Salad

Preparation Time: 10 minutes | Cooking Time: 45 minutes | Portion Size: 4 servings | Difficulty Level: Medium

Ingredients:

- 4 medium beets, scrubbed and trimmed
- 4 cups mixed greens (arugula, spinach, or lettuce)
- ½ cup crumbled goat cheese
- ¼ cup walnuts, chopped
- 2 tablespoons fresh parsley, chopped
- Salt and pepper to taste

Dressing:

- 2 tablespoons balsamic vinegar
- 1 tablespoon lemon juice
- 2 teaspoons honey
- ¼ cup olive oil
- Salt and pepper to taste

Instructions:

1. **Roast the Beets:**

1. Preheat the oven to 400°F (200°C).

2. Wrap each beet individually in aluminum foil and place them on a baking sheet.

3. Roast for 45 minutes to 1 hour, or until the beets are tender when pierced with a fork.

4. Allow the beets to cool, then peel and dice them into bite-sized pieces.

2. **Prepare the Dressing:**

   1. In a small bowl, whisk together balsamic vinegar, lemon juice, honey, olive oil, salt, and pepper.

3. **Assemble the Salad:**

   1. In a large bowl, toss the mixed greens with half of the dressing.

2. Divide the greens among four plates.

3. Top each plate with roasted beets, crumbled goat cheese, chopped walnuts, and parsley.

4. Drizzle with the remaining dressing.

5. Season with salt and pepper to taste.

6. Serve immediately and enjoy!

Nutritional Information (per serving):

Total Carbohydrates: 22g | **Fiber:** 5g | **Sugars:** 15g | **Protein:** 7g | **Total Fat:** 14g | **Saturated Fat:** 3g | **Calories:** 230 | **Sodium:** 160mg | **Calcium:** 80mg | **Iron:** 1.5mg

Vegetable and Bean Chili

Preparation Time: 15 minutes | Cooking Time: 35 minutes | Portion Size: 4 servings | Difficulty Level: Medium

Ingredients:

- 2 tablespoons olive oil
- 1 onion, diced
- 2 cloves garlic, minced
- 1 red bell pepper, diced
- 1 green bell pepper, diced
- 1 zucchini, diced
- 1 carrot, diced
- 1 can (15 ounces) black beans, drained and rinsed
- 1 can (15 ounces) kidney beans, drained and rinsed
- 1 can (15 ounces) diced tomatoes
- 1 cup vegetable broth
- 2 tablespoons tomato paste
- 1 tablespoon chili powder
- 1 teaspoon cumin
- 1 teaspoon smoked paprika
- 1 teaspoon oregano
- Salt and pepper to taste
- Fresh cilantro, chopped (for garnish)
- Low-fat Greek yogurt (for serving)

Instructions:

1. **Sauté the Vegetables:**

    1. In a large pot, heat olive oil over medium heat.

    2. Add onion and garlic, and sauté for 3-4 minutes until softened.

    3. Add red bell pepper, green bell pepper, zucchini, and carrot, and sauté for another 5 minutes.

2. **Make the Chili:**

    1. Stir in black beans, kidney beans, diced tomatoes, vegetable broth, and tomato paste.

    2. Add chili powder, cumin, smoked paprika, oregano, salt, and pepper.

3. Bring to a boil, then reduce heat to low and simmer for 20-25 minutes, stirring occasionally.

3. **Serve:**

    1. Ladle the chili into bowls and garnish with chopped cilantro.

    2. Top with a dollop of low-fat Greek yogurt.

    3. Serve immediately and enjoy!

Nutritional Information (per serving):

Total Carbohydrates: 40g | **Fiber:** 12g | **Sugars:** 9g | **Protein:** 13g | **Total Fat:** 8g | **Saturated Fat:** 1g | **Calories:** 250 | **Sodium:** 380mg | **Calcium:** 100mg | **Iron:** 4mg

Baked Tilapia with Mango Salsa

Preparation Time: 10 minutes | Cooking Time: 15 minutes | Portion Size: 4 servings | Difficulty Level: Easy

Ingredients:

Baked Tilapia:

- 4 tilapia fillets (6 ounces each)
- 1 tablespoon olive oil
- 1 teaspoon smoked paprika
- 1 teaspoon garlic powder
- ½ teaspoon cumin
- Salt and pepper to taste
- Lemon wedges (for serving)

Mango Salsa:

- 1 ripe mango, diced
- ½ red bell pepper, diced
- ¼ cup red onion, finely chopped
- ¼ cup fresh cilantro, chopped
- 2 tablespoons lime juice
- 1 teaspoon olive oil
- Salt and pepper to taste

Instructions:

1. **Prepare the Mango Salsa:**

    1. In a medium bowl, combine diced mango, red bell pepper, red onion, cilantro, lime juice, olive oil, salt, and pepper.

    2. Mix well and set aside.

2. **Prepare the Tilapia:**

    1. Preheat the oven to 400°F (200°C).

    2. Place the tilapia fillets on a baking sheet lined with parchment paper.

    3. Drizzle each fillet with olive oil and season with smoked paprika, garlic powder, cumin, salt, and pepper.

    4. Bake in the preheated oven for 12-15 minutes, or until the tilapia is

cooked through and flakes easily with a fork.

3. **Serve:**

    1. Place each tilapia fillet on a plate and top with mango salsa.

    2. Garnish with lemon wedges and serve immediately.

Nutritional Information (per serving):

Total Carbohydrates: 10g | **Fiber:** 2g | **Sugars:** 6g | **Protein:** 26g | **Total Fat:** 8g | **Saturated Fat:** 1.5g | **Calories:** 190 | **Sodium:** 230mg | **Calcium:** 40mg | **Iron:** 1mg

Asian Chicken Salad with Low-Sodium Soy Dressing

Preparation Time: 15 minutes | Cooking Time: 10 minutes | Portion Size: 4 servings | Difficulty Level: Easy

Ingredients:

Salad:

- 1 pound boneless, skinless chicken breasts
- 1 tablespoon olive oil
- Salt and pepper to taste
- 4 cups mixed greens
- 1 cup shredded red cabbage
- 1 cup shredded carrots
- 1 cucumber, thinly sliced
- ½ cup edamame beans, shelled
- 2 green onions, chopped
- 2 tablespoons sesame seeds

Low-Sodium Soy Dressing:

- 3 tablespoons low-sodium soy sauce
- 2 tablespoons rice vinegar
- 1 tablespoon sesame oil
- 1 tablespoon honey
- 1 teaspoon grated ginger
- 1 teaspoon lime juice

Instructions:

1. **Cook the Chicken:**

    1. In a large skillet, heat olive oil over medium-high heat.

    2. Season the chicken breasts with salt and pepper.

    3. Add the chicken breasts to the skillet and cook for 5-6 minutes on each side, or until fully cooked.

    4. Remove from the skillet, let cool slightly, and slice into strips.

2. **Prepare the Dressing:**

    1. In a small bowl, whisk together soy sauce, rice vinegar, sesame oil, honey, grated ginger, and lime juice.

    2. Set aside.

3. **Assemble the Salad:**

    1. In a large bowl, combine mixed greens, shredded red cabbage, shredded carrots, cucumber, edamame beans, and green onions.

    2. Divide the salad evenly among four plates.

    3. Top each plate with sliced chicken and sesame seeds.

4. Drizzle with the low-sodium soy dressing.

4. **Serve:**

    1. Serve immediately and enjoy!

Nutritional Information (per serving):

Total Carbohydrates: 14g | **Fiber:** 4g | **Sugars:** 7g | **Protein:** 24g | **Total Fat:** 10g | **Saturated Fat:** 1.5g | **Calories:** 240 | **Sodium:** 350mg | **Calcium:** 50mg | **Iron:** 2mg

Stuffed Acorn Squash with Quinoa and Cranberries

Preparation Time: 15 minutes | Cooking Time: 45 minutes | Portion Size: 4 servings | Difficulty Level: Medium

Ingredients:

- 2 medium acorn squashes, halved and seeds removed
- 1 tablespoon olive oil
- 1 cup quinoa, rinsed
- 2 cups vegetable broth
- 1 small onion, diced
- 2 cloves garlic, minced
- ½ cup dried cranberries
- ¼ cup walnuts, chopped
- 2 tablespoons fresh parsley, chopped
- 1 teaspoon ground cinnamon
- ½ teaspoon ground nutmeg
- Salt and pepper to taste

Instructions:

1. **Roast the Acorn Squash:**

    1. Preheat the oven to 400°F (200°C).

    2. Rub the inside of each acorn squash half with olive oil and season with salt and pepper.

    3. Place the squash halves cut side down on a baking sheet lined with parchment paper.

    4. Roast for 30-35 minutes, or until the squash is tender when pierced with a fork.

2. **Prepare the Quinoa Filling:**

    1. In a medium saucepan, bring vegetable broth to a boil. Add quinoa, reduce heat to low, cover, and simmer for 15 minutes, or until the liquid is absorbed.

    2. In a skillet, heat olive oil over medium heat. Add onion and garlic, and sauté for 3-4 minutes until softened.

    3. Stir in cooked quinoa, dried cranberries, walnuts, parsley, cinnamon, nutmeg, salt, and pepper.

    4. Cook for another 2-3 minutes until heated through.

3. **Stuff the Acorn Squash:**

    1. Remove the roasted acorn squash halves from the oven and flip them over.

    2. Divide the quinoa filling evenly among the squash halves.

3. Return to the oven and bake for an additional 10 minutes.

4. **Serve:**

   1. Garnish with additional parsley if desired.

   2. Serve immediately and enjoy!

Southwest Chicken Bowl with Brown Rice and Black Beans

Preparation Time: 15 minutes | Cooking Time: 25 minutes | Portion Size: 4 servings | Difficulty Level: Medium

Ingredients:

Chicken Marinade:

- 1 pound boneless, skinless chicken breast, cut into strips
- 1 tablespoon olive oil
- 1 teaspoon cumin
- 1 teaspoon smoked paprika
- 1 teaspoon chili powder
- ½ teaspoon garlic powder
- ½ teaspoon onion powder
- Salt and pepper to taste

Brown Rice:

- 1 cup brown rice, rinsed
- 2 cups water

Southwest Bowl:

- 1 can (15 ounces) black beans, drained and rinsed
- 1 cup corn kernels (fresh, frozen, or canned)
- 1 red bell pepper, diced
- 1 avocado, diced
- 2 cups mixed greens
- ¼ cup fresh cilantro, chopped
- Lime wedges (for serving)

Dressing:

- ¼ cup Greek yogurt
- 2 tablespoons lime juice
- 1 tablespoon olive oil
- 1 teaspoon cumin
- Salt and pepper to taste

Instructions:

1. **Marinate the Chicken:**

   1. In a medium bowl, combine olive oil, cumin, smoked paprika, chili powder, garlic powder, onion powder, salt, and pepper.

   2. Add the chicken strips and toss to coat evenly.

   3. Cover and marinate for at least 15 minutes.

2. **Cook the Brown Rice:**

   1. In a medium saucepan, bring 2 cups of water to a boil.

   2. Add the rinsed brown rice, reduce heat to low, cover, and simmer for

Nutritional Information (per serving):

Total Carbohydrates: 50g | **Fiber:** 8g | **Sugars:** 14g | **Protein:** 8g | **Total Fat:** 10g | **Saturated Fat:** 1g | **Calories:** 320 | **Sodium:** 180mg | **Calcium:** 80mg | **Iron:** 2.5mg

25 minutes or until the water is absorbed.

   3. Remove from heat and let sit for 5 minutes, then fluff with a fork.

3. **Cook the Chicken:**

   1. In a large skillet, heat 1 tablespoon of olive oil over medium-high heat.

   2. Add the marinated chicken strips and cook for 5-7 minutes until fully cooked and no longer pink.

   3. Remove from the skillet and set aside.

4. **Prepare the Dressing:**

   1. In a small bowl, whisk together Greek yogurt, lime juice, olive oil, cumin, salt, and pepper.

5. **Assemble the Southwest Bowl:**

   1. Divide the cooked brown rice evenly among four bowls.

   2. Top each bowl with black beans, corn, red bell pepper, avocado, mixed greens, and cooked chicken strips.

   3. Drizzle with the dressing and garnish with fresh cilantro and lime wedges.

6. **Serve:**

   1. Serve immediately and enjoy!

Nutritional Information (per serving):

Total Carbohydrates: 45g | **Fiber:** 9g | **Sugars:** 5g | **Protein:** 28g | **Total Fat:** 12g | **Saturated Fat:** 2g | **Calories:** 420 | **Sodium:** 420mg | **Calcium:** 90mg | **Iron:** 3mg

Broccoli and Cheese Stuffed Chicken Breast

Preparation Time: 15 minutes | Cooking Time: 30 minutes | Portion Size: 4 servings | Difficulty Level: Medium

Ingredients:

- 4 boneless, skinless chicken breasts
- 1 cup broccoli florets, finely chopped
- ½ cup shredded low-fat cheddar cheese
- ¼ cup low-fat cream cheese, softened
- 1 tablespoon Parmesan cheese, grated
- 1 tablespoon Dijon mustard
- 1 teaspoon garlic powder
- 1 teaspoon onion powder
- 1 teaspoon smoked paprika
- Salt and pepper to taste
- 1 tablespoon olive oil

Instructions:

1. **Prepare the Chicken:**

   1. Preheat the oven to 375°F (190°C).

   2. Place the chicken breasts on a cutting board. Use a sharp knife to cut a pocket into the side of each breast without cutting all the way through.

2. **Prepare the Filling:**

   1. In a medium bowl, combine broccoli florets, cheddar cheese, cream cheese, Parmesan cheese, Dijon mustard, garlic powder, onion powder, salt, and pepper.

3. **Stuff the Chicken:**

1. Spoon the broccoli and cheese mixture into the pockets of each chicken breast.

2. Secure with toothpicks if needed.

4. Cook the Chicken:

1. In a large oven-safe skillet, heat olive oil over medium-high heat.

2. Add the stuffed chicken breasts and sear for 3-4 minutes on each side until golden brown.

3. Sprinkle smoked paprika over the chicken breasts.

4. Transfer the skillet to the preheated oven and bake for 20-25 minutes or until the chicken is fully cooked and no longer pink.

5. Serve:

1. Remove the toothpicks from the chicken breasts.

2. Serve immediately and enjoy!

Nutritional Information (per serving):

Total Carbohydrates: 5g | **Fiber:** 2g | **Sugars:** 1g | **Protein:** 30g | **Total Fat:** 10g | **Saturated Fat:** 3.5g | **Calories:** 230 | **Sodium:** 300mg | **Calcium:** 100mg | **Iron:** 1mg

Mediterranean Tuna Salad with Mixed Greens

Preparation Time: 10 minutes | Cooking Time: 0 minutes | Portion Size: 4 servings | Difficulty Level: Easy

Ingredients:

- 2 cans (5 ounces each) tuna in water, drained
- 4 cups mixed greens (arugula, spinach, lettuce)
- 1 cucumber, diced
- 1 cup cherry tomatoes, halved
- ½ cup Kalamata olives, pitted and sliced
- ½ cup crumbled feta cheese
- ¼ cup red onion, thinly sliced
- 2 tablespoons capers, rinsed and drained
- 2 tablespoons fresh parsley, chopped

Dressing:

- 3 tablespoons olive oil
- 2 tablespoons lemon juice
- 1 teaspoon Dijon mustard
- 1 teaspoon oregano
- Salt and pepper to taste

Instructions:

1. **Prepare the Dressing:**

    1. In a small bowl, whisk together olive oil, lemon juice, Dijon mustard, oregano, salt, and pepper.

    2. Set aside.

2. **Assemble the Salad:**

    1. In a large bowl, combine mixed greens, cucumber, cherry tomatoes, Kalamata olives, feta cheese, red onion, capers, and parsley.

    2. Add the drained tuna and toss gently to combine.

3. **Dress the Salad:**

    1. Pour the dressing over the salad and toss gently to coat.

    2. Divide the salad evenly among four plates.

4. **Serve:**

    1. Serve immediately and enjoy!

Nutritional Information (per serving):

Total Carbohydrates: 8g | **Fiber:** 3g | **Sugars:** 4g | **Protein:** 24g | **Total Fat:** 14g | **Saturated Fat:** 3g | **Calories:** 240 | **Sodium:** 380mg | **Calcium:** 120mg | **Iron:** 2mg

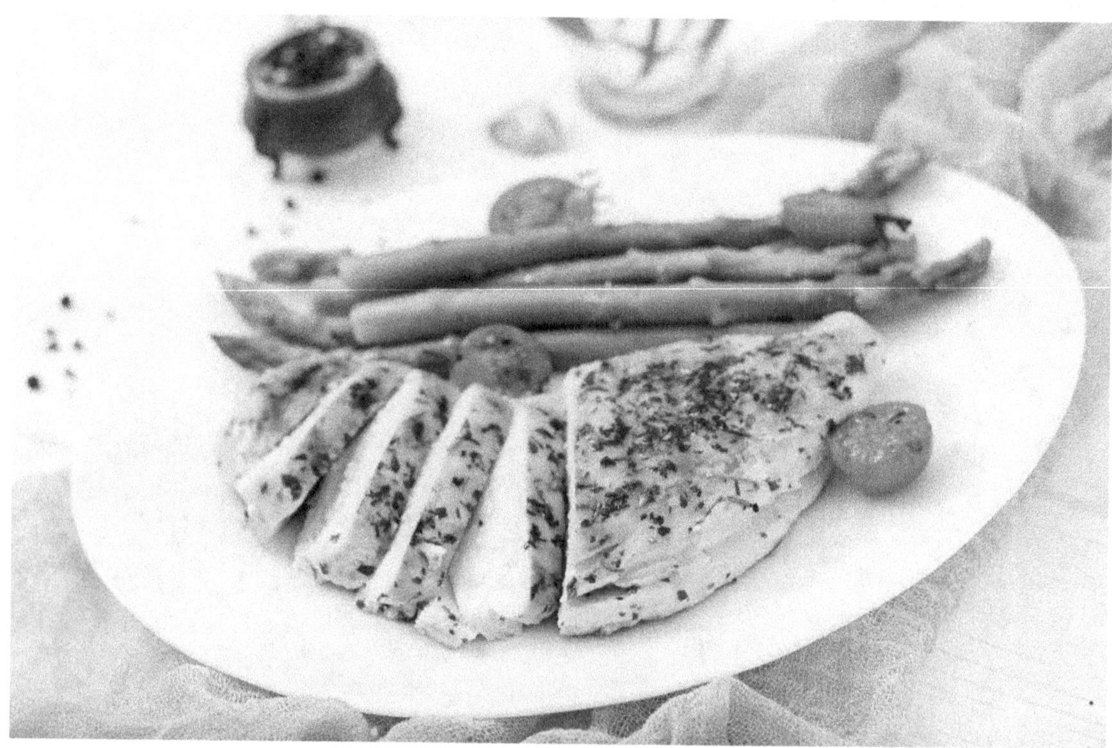

Herb-Roasted Chicken Breast with Steamed Asparagus

Preparation Time: 10 minutes | Cooking Time: 20 minutes | Portion Size: 4 servings | Difficulty Level: Easy

Ingredients:

Herb-Roasted Chicken:

- 4 boneless, skinless chicken breasts
- 2 tablespoons olive oil
- 1 teaspoon garlic powder
- 1 teaspoon onion powder
- 1 teaspoon dried thyme
- 1 teaspoon dried rosemary
- ½ teaspoon smoked paprika
- Salt and pepper to taste
- Lemon wedges (for serving)

Steamed Asparagus:

- 1 pound asparagus, trimmed
- 1 tablespoon olive oil
- 1 teaspoon lemon zest
- Salt and pepper to taste

Instructions:

1. **Prepare the Chicken:**

    1. Preheat the oven to 400°F (200°C).

    2. In a small bowl, mix together olive oil, garlic powder, onion powder, thyme, rosemary, smoked paprika, salt, and pepper.

3. Rub the spice mixture over the chicken breasts, ensuring they are evenly coated.

2. **Roast the Chicken:**

   1. Place the chicken breasts on a baking sheet lined with parchment paper.

   2. Roast for 18-20 minutes, or until the chicken is fully cooked and no longer pink in the center.

   3. Remove from the oven and let rest for 5 minutes before slicing.

3. **Steam the Asparagus:**

   1. While the chicken is roasting, bring a pot of water to a boil and place a steamer basket over it.

   2. Add the asparagus to the steamer basket, cover, and steam for 5-6 minutes until tender-crisp.

   3. Remove the asparagus from the steamer and toss with olive oil, lemon zest, salt, and pepper.

4. **Serve:**

   1. Divide the roasted chicken breasts and steamed asparagus evenly among four plates.

   2. Serve with lemon wedges and enjoy immediately!

Nutritional Information (per serving):

Total Carbohydrates: 6g | **Fiber:** 3g | **Sugars:** 2g | **Protein:** 30g | **Total Fat:** 12g | **Saturated Fat:** 2g | **Calories:** 240 | **Sodium:** 220mg | **Calcium:** 50mg | **Iron:** 2mg

Pork Tenderloin with Apple Cider Reduction

Preparation Time: 15 minutes | Cooking Time: 30 minutes | Portion Size: 4 servings | Difficulty Level: Medium

Ingredients:

Pork Tenderloin:

- 1 pound pork tenderloin, trimmed
- 2 tablespoons olive oil
- 1 teaspoon garlic powder
- 1 teaspoon smoked paprika
- 1 teaspoon thyme
- Salt and pepper to taste

Apple Cider Reduction:

- 1 cup apple cider
- 2 tablespoons apple cider vinegar
- 1 tablespoon Dijon mustard
- 1 tablespoon honey
- 1 tablespoon unsalted butter
- 1 teaspoon cornstarch
- Salt and pepper to taste
- Fresh parsley, chopped (for garnish)

Instructions:

1. **Prepare and Sear the Pork Tenderloin:**

   1. Preheat the oven to 400°F (200°C).

   2. In a small bowl, mix together olive oil, garlic powder, smoked paprika, thyme, salt, and pepper.

   3. Rub the spice mixture over the pork tenderloin.

   4. In a large oven-safe skillet, heat 1 tablespoon of olive oil over medium-high heat.

5. Sear the pork tenderloin on all sides until golden brown, about 4-5 minutes per side.

6. Transfer the skillet to the preheated oven and roast for 15-20 minutes, or until the internal temperature reaches 145°F (63°C).

7. Remove from the oven and let rest for 5 minutes before slicing.

2. **Prepare the Apple Cider Reduction:**

1. In a medium saucepan, bring apple cider and apple cider vinegar to a boil over medium heat.

2. Reduce the heat to low and simmer for 10 minutes until the liquid has reduced by half.

3. Stir in Dijon mustard, honey, butter, cornstarch, salt, and pepper.

4. Continue to simmer for another 2-3 minutes until the sauce thickens.

3. **Serve:**

1. Slice the pork tenderloin into medallions and arrange on a serving plate.

2. Drizzle the apple cider reduction over the pork and garnish with chopped parsley.

3. Serve immediately and enjoy!

Nutritional Information (per serving):

Total Carbohydrates: 10g | **Fiber:** 1g | **Sugars:** 8g | **Protein:** 28g | **Total Fat:** 8g | **Saturated Fat:** 2g | **Calories:** 220 | **Sodium:** 220mg | **Calcium:** 30mg | **Iron:** 2mg

Vegetable Lasagna with Low-Fat Ricotta and Spinach

Preparation Time: 20 minutes | Cooking Time: 45 minutes | Portion Size: 4 servings | Difficulty Level: Medium

Ingredients:

Lasagna:

- 9 lasagna noodles, cooked and drained
- 2 cups low-fat ricotta cheese
- 2 cups fresh spinach, chopped
- 2 cups shredded low-fat mozzarella cheese
- 1 cup grated Parmesan cheese
- 1 egg, beaten
- 1 zucchini, diced
- 1 yellow squash, diced
- 1 red bell pepper, diced
- 1 cup mushrooms, sliced
- 2 cloves garlic, minced
- 2 tablespoons olive oil
- Salt and pepper to taste

Tomato Sauce:

- 2 tablespoons olive oil
- 1 onion, diced
- 2 cloves garlic, minced
- 1 can (28 ounces) crushed tomatoes
- 1 teaspoon oregano
- 1 teaspoon basil
- 1 teaspoon thyme
- Salt and pepper to taste

Instructions:

1. **Prepare the Tomato Sauce:**

   1. In a medium saucepan, heat olive oil over medium heat.

   2. Add onion and garlic, and sauté for 3-4 minutes until softened.

   3. Stir in crushed tomatoes, oregano, basil, thyme, salt, and pepper.

   4. Bring to a simmer and cook for 15 minutes, stirring occasionally.

   5. Set aside.

2. **Prepare the Vegetable Filling:**

   1. In a large skillet, heat olive oil over medium heat.

   2. Add zucchini, yellow squash, red bell pepper, mushrooms, and garlic.

   3. Sauté for 5-6 minutes until the vegetables are tender.

   4. Season with salt and pepper, and set aside.

3. **Prepare the Ricotta Mixture:**

   1. In a medium bowl, combine low-fat ricotta cheese, chopped spinach, beaten egg, salt, and pepper.

   2. Mix well and set aside.

4. **Assemble the Lasagna:**

   1. Preheat the oven to 375°F (190°C).

   2. In a 9x13-inch baking dish, spread a layer of tomato sauce.

   3. Place three lasagna noodles over the sauce.

   4. Spread a layer of the ricotta mixture over the noodles.

   5. Add a layer of the sautéed vegetables and sprinkle with mozzarella cheese.

   6. Repeat layers twice more, ending with a layer of tomato sauce on top.

   7. Sprinkle with grated Parmesan cheese.

5. **Bake the Lasagna:**

   1. Cover the baking dish with foil and bake for 30 minutes.

   2. Remove the foil and bake for another 10-15 minutes until the cheese is melted and bubbly.

   3. Let the lasagna cool for 10 minutes before serving.

6. **Serve:**

   1. Slice the lasagna into portions and serve immediately.

Nutritional Information (per serving):

Total Carbohydrates: 45g | **Fiber:** 7g | **Sugars:** 12g | **Protein:** 22g | **Total Fat:** 12g | **Saturated Fat:** 5g | **Calories:** 360 | **Sodium:** 450mg | **Calcium:** 350mg | **Iron:** 4mg

Grilled Tilapia with Lemon Herb Quinoa

Preparation Time: 10 minutes | Cooking Time: 20 minutes | Portion Size: 4 servings | Difficulty Level: Easy

Ingredients:

Grilled Tilapia:

- 4 tilapia fillets (6 ounces each)

- 2 tablespoons olive oil

- 1 teaspoon smoked paprika

- 1 teaspoon garlic powder
- 1 teaspoon onion powder
- ½ teaspoon cumin
- Salt and pepper to taste
- Lemon wedges (for serving)

Lemon Herb Quinoa:

- 1 cup quinoa, rinsed
- 2 cups low-sodium vegetable broth
- 2 tablespoons lemon juice
- 1 teaspoon lemon zest
- 2 tablespoons fresh parsley, chopped
- 2 tablespoons fresh basil, chopped
- Salt and pepper to taste

Instructions:

1. **Prepare the Grilled Tilapia:**
   1. Preheat the grill to medium-high heat.
   2. In a small bowl, mix together olive oil, smoked paprika, garlic powder, onion powder, cumin, salt, and pepper.
   3. Rub the spice mixture over the tilapia fillets.
   4. Lightly oil the grill grates or use a grilling basket.
   5. Grill the tilapia fillets for 3-4 minutes per side or until fully cooked and the fish flakes easily with a fork.

2. **Prepare the Lemon Herb Quinoa:**
   1. In a medium saucepan, bring vegetable broth to a boil.
   2. Add the rinsed quinoa, reduce heat to low, cover, and simmer for 15 minutes or until the broth is absorbed.
   3. Fluff the quinoa with a fork and stir in lemon juice, lemon zest, parsley, basil, salt, and pepper.

3. **Serve:**
   1. Divide the lemon herb quinoa evenly among four plates.
   2. Place a grilled tilapia fillet on top of each plate of quinoa.
   3. Garnish with lemon wedges and serve immediately.

Nutritional Information (per serving):

Total Carbohydrates: 28g | **Fiber:** 4g | **Sugars:** 2g | **Protein:** 30g | **Total Fat:** 12g | **Saturated Fat:** 2g | **Calories:** 330 | **Sodium:** 300mg | **Calcium:** 60mg | **Iron:** 3mg

Beef Stir-Fry with Broccoli and Bell Pepper

Preparation Time: 10 minutes | Cooking Time: 15 minutes | Portion Size: 4 servings | Difficulty Level: Medium

Ingredients:

Beef Marinade:

- 1 pound flank steak, sliced thinly against the grain
- 2 tablespoons soy sauce (low-sodium)
- 1 tablespoon rice vinegar
- 1 tablespoon cornstarch
- 1 teaspoon sesame oil

- 1 teaspoon grated ginger

Stir-Fry Sauce:

- ¼ cup soy sauce (low-sodium)
- 2 tablespoons hoisin sauce
- 2 tablespoons oyster sauce
- 1 tablespoon honey
- 1 tablespoon rice vinegar
- 1 teaspoon sesame oil
- 1 teaspoon cornstarch

Stir-Fry:

- 2 tablespoons vegetable oil
- 2 cloves garlic, minced
- 1 tablespoon grated ginger
- 1 broccoli crown, cut into florets
- 1 red bell pepper, sliced thinly
- 1 yellow bell pepper, sliced thinly
- 2 green onions, chopped (for garnish)
- Sesame seeds (for garnish)

Instructions:

1. **Marinate the Beef:**

   1. In a medium bowl, whisk together soy sauce, rice vinegar, cornstarch, sesame oil, and grated ginger.

   2. Add sliced flank steak to the bowl and toss to coat evenly.

   3. Let marinate for at least 15 minutes.

2. **Prepare the Stir-Fry Sauce:**

   1. In a small bowl, whisk together soy sauce, hoisin sauce, oyster sauce, honey, rice vinegar, sesame oil, and cornstarch.

   2. Set aside.

3. **Cook the Stir-Fry:**

   1. In a large skillet or wok, heat 1 tablespoon of vegetable oil over high heat.

   2. Add marinated beef and stir-fry for 2-3 minutes until just cooked. Remove the beef from the skillet and set aside.

   3. In the same skillet, add the remaining vegetable oil, garlic, and grated ginger, and stir-fry for 30 seconds until fragrant.

   4. Add broccoli florets and stir-fry for 2-3 minutes.

   5. Add red and yellow bell peppers and stir-fry for another 2 minutes.

4. **Combine and Serve:**

   1. Return the beef to the skillet, add the stir-fry sauce, and stir-fry for another 2-3 minutes until the sauce thickens.

   2. Garnish with chopped green onions and sesame seeds.

   3. Serve immediately and enjoy!

Nutritional Information (per serving):

Total Carbohydrates: 15g | **Fiber:** 4g | **Sugars:** 6g | **Protein:** 24g | **Total Fat:** 14g | **Saturated Fat:** 4g | **Calories:** 290 | **Sodium:** 590mg | **Calcium:** 60mg | **Iron:** 3mg

Butternut Squash Risotto

Preparation Time: 10 minutes | Cooking Time: 30 minutes | Portion Size: 4 servings | Difficulty Level: Medium

Ingredients:

- 1 tablespoon olive oil
- 1 small onion, diced
- 2 cloves garlic, minced
- 1 cup Arborio rice
- 1 cup butternut squash, peeled and diced
- 4 cups low-sodium vegetable broth, warmed
- ½ cup dry white wine (optional)
- 1 teaspoon thyme
- ½ teaspoon sage
- Salt and pepper to taste
- ½ cup grated Parmesan cheese
- 2 tablespoons unsalted butter
- Fresh parsley, chopped (for garnish)

Instructions:

1. **Sauté Aromatics:**

   1. In a large skillet or saucepan, heat olive oil over medium heat.
   2. Add onion and garlic, and sauté for 3-4 minutes until softened.

2. **Prepare the Risotto Base:**

   1. Add Arborio rice to the skillet and stir to coat with the oil.
   2. Add butternut squash and cook for 2-3 minutes, stirring occasionally.
   3. Stir in white wine (if using) and cook until the liquid is mostly absorbed.

3. **Cook the Risotto:**

   1. Add 1 cup of warm vegetable broth to the skillet and stir continuously until the liquid is absorbed.
   2. Continue adding broth, 1 cup at a time, stirring constantly until the liquid is absorbed before adding more.
   3. Repeat until all the broth is used and the rice is creamy and cooked through.
   4. Stir in thyme, sage, salt, and pepper.

4. **Finish the Risotto:**

   1. Remove the skillet from heat and stir in Parmesan cheese and butter.
   2. Adjust seasoning with salt and pepper to taste.

5. **Serve:**

   1. Divide the risotto evenly among four plates.
   2. Garnish with chopped parsley and serve immediately.

Nutritional Information (per serving):

Total Carbohydrates: 50g | **Fiber:** 4g | **Sugars:** 4g | **Protein:** 10g | **Total Fat:** 12g | **Saturated Fat:** 5g | **Calories:** 350 | **Sodium:** 340mg | **Calcium:** 150mg | **Iron:** 2mg

Baked Cod with Olive Tapenade

Preparation Time: 15 minutes | Cooking Time: 15 minutes | Portion Size: 4 servings | Difficulty Level: Easy

Ingredients:

Baked Cod:

- 4 cod fillets (6 ounces each)
- 2 tablespoons olive oil
- 1 teaspoon smoked paprika
- 1 teaspoon garlic powder
- ½ teaspoon onion powder
- Salt and pepper to taste
- Lemon wedges (for serving)

Olive Tapenade:

- ½ cup Kalamata olives, pitted and chopped
- ¼ cup green olives, pitted and chopped
- 2 tablespoons capers, rinsed and drained
- 2 tablespoons fresh parsley, chopped
- 1 tablespoon lemon juice
- 1 tablespoon olive oil
- 1 clove garlic, minced
- Salt and pepper to taste

Instructions:

1. **Prepare the Olive Tapenade:**
   1. In a medium bowl, combine Kalamata olives, green olives, capers, parsley, lemon juice, olive oil, garlic, salt, and pepper.
   2. Mix well and set aside.
2. **Prepare the Baked Cod:**
   1. Preheat the oven to 400°F (200°C).
   2. In a small bowl, mix together olive oil, smoked paprika, garlic powder, onion powder, salt, and pepper.
   3. Rub the spice mixture over the cod fillets.
   4. Place the cod fillets on a baking sheet lined with parchment paper.
   5. Bake in the preheated oven for 12-15 minutes, or until the fish is fully cooked and flakes easily with a fork.
3. **Serve:**
   1. Place each cod fillet on a plate and spoon the olive tapenade over the top.
   2. Serve with lemon wedges and enjoy immediately!

Nutritional Information (per serving):

Total Carbohydrates: 4g | **Fiber:** 1g | **Sugars:** 1g | **Protein:** 25g | **Total Fat:** 10g | **Saturated Fat:** 2g | **Calories:** 210 | **Sodium:** 350mg | **Calcium:** 50mg | **Iron:** 1.5mg

Turkey Meatloaf with Sweet Potato Mash

Preparation Time: 20 minutes | Cooking Time: 50 minutes | Portion Size: 4 servings | Difficulty Level: Medium

Ingredients:

Turkey Meatloaf:

- 1 pound ground turkey
- 1 small onion, diced
- 2 cloves garlic, minced
- 1 egg, beaten
- ½ cup breadcrumbs
- ¼ cup low-fat milk
- 2 tablespoons ketchup
- 2 tablespoons Worcestershire sauce
- 1 tablespoon Dijon mustard
- 1 teaspoon thyme
- 1 teaspoon smoked paprika
- Salt and pepper to taste
- ¼ cup ketchup (for glaze)

Sweet Potato Mash:

- 2 large sweet potatoes, peeled and diced
- 2 tablespoons unsalted butter
- ¼ cup low-fat milk
- Salt and pepper to taste

Instructions:

1. **Prepare the Turkey Meatloaf:**
    1. Preheat the oven to 375°F (190°C).
    2. In a large bowl, combine ground turkey, onion, garlic, beaten egg, breadcrumbs, milk, ketchup, Worcestershire sauce, Dijon mustard, thyme, smoked paprika, salt, and pepper.
    3. Mix until well combined.
    4. Transfer the mixture to a loaf pan and shape it into a loaf.
    5. Spread ¼ cup of ketchup over the top as a glaze.
    6. Bake for 45-50 minutes, or until the internal temperature reaches 165°F (74°C).
    7. Remove from the oven and let rest for 10 minutes before slicing.

2. **Prepare the Sweet Potato Mash:**
    1. While the meatloaf is baking, bring a pot of water to a boil.
    2. Add diced sweet potatoes and boil for 15-20 minutes until tender.
    3. Drain and return the sweet potatoes to the pot.
    4. Add butter, milk, salt, and pepper.
    5. Mash until smooth and creamy.

3. **Serve:**
    1. Slice the turkey meatloaf and serve with a generous portion of sweet potato mash.
    2. Enjoy immediately!

Nutritional Information (per serving):

Total Carbohydrates: 37g | **Fiber:** 5g | **Sugars:** 12g | **Protein:** 27g | **Total Fat:** 12g | **Saturated Fat:** 4g | **Calories:** 360 | **Sodium:** 540mg | **Calcium:** 90mg | **Iron:** 2.5mg

Vegetarian Paella with Saffron and Mixed Vegetables

Preparation Time: 15 minutes | Cooking Time: 35 minutes | Portion Size: 4 servings | Difficulty Level: Medium

Ingredients:

- 2 tablespoons olive oil
- 1 onion, diced
- 2 cloves garlic, minced
- 1 bell pepper, diced
- 1 zucchini, diced
- 1 cup green beans, trimmed and cut into 1-inch pieces
- 1 cup cherry tomatoes, halved
- 1 cup frozen peas
- 1 cup Arborio rice (or Bomba rice, if available)
- 4 cups low-sodium vegetable broth, warmed
- ½ cup white wine (optional)
- 1 teaspoon smoked paprika
- 1 teaspoon thyme
- ½ teaspoon saffron threads, soaked in 2 tablespoons warm water
- Salt and pepper to taste
- 1 lemon, cut into wedges
- Fresh parsley, chopped (for garnish)

Instructions:

1. **Sauté Aromatics and Vegetables:**
   1. In a large skillet or paella pan, heat olive oil over medium heat.
   2. Add onion and garlic, and sauté for 3-4 minutes until softened.
   3. Add bell pepper, zucchini, and green beans, and sauté for another 5 minutes until slightly tender.

2. **Prepare the Paella Base:**
   1. Stir in Arborio rice, smoked paprika, thyme, and saffron threads (including soaking liquid).
   2. Cook for 2-3 minutes, stirring constantly, until the rice is well coated with oil and spices.

3. **Cook the Paella:**
   1. Pour in white wine (if using) and cook until mostly absorbed.
   2. Add warmed vegetable broth, 1 cup at a time, stirring occasionally and allowing the liquid to be absorbed before adding more.
   3. Stir in cherry tomatoes and frozen peas.
   4. Season with salt and pepper to taste.
   5. Reduce the heat to low and let the paella simmer for 20-25 minutes, stirring occasionally until the rice is cooked and the liquid is absorbed.

4. **Serve:**
   1. Garnish the paella with lemon wedges and chopped parsley.
   2. Serve immediately and enjoy!

Nutritional Information (per serving):

Total Carbohydrates: 50g | **Fiber:** 6g | **Sugars:** 7g | **Protein:** 8g | **Total Fat:** 10g | **Saturated Fat:** 1.5g | **Calories:** 310 | **Sodium:** 360mg | **Calcium:** 60mg | **Iron:** 3mg

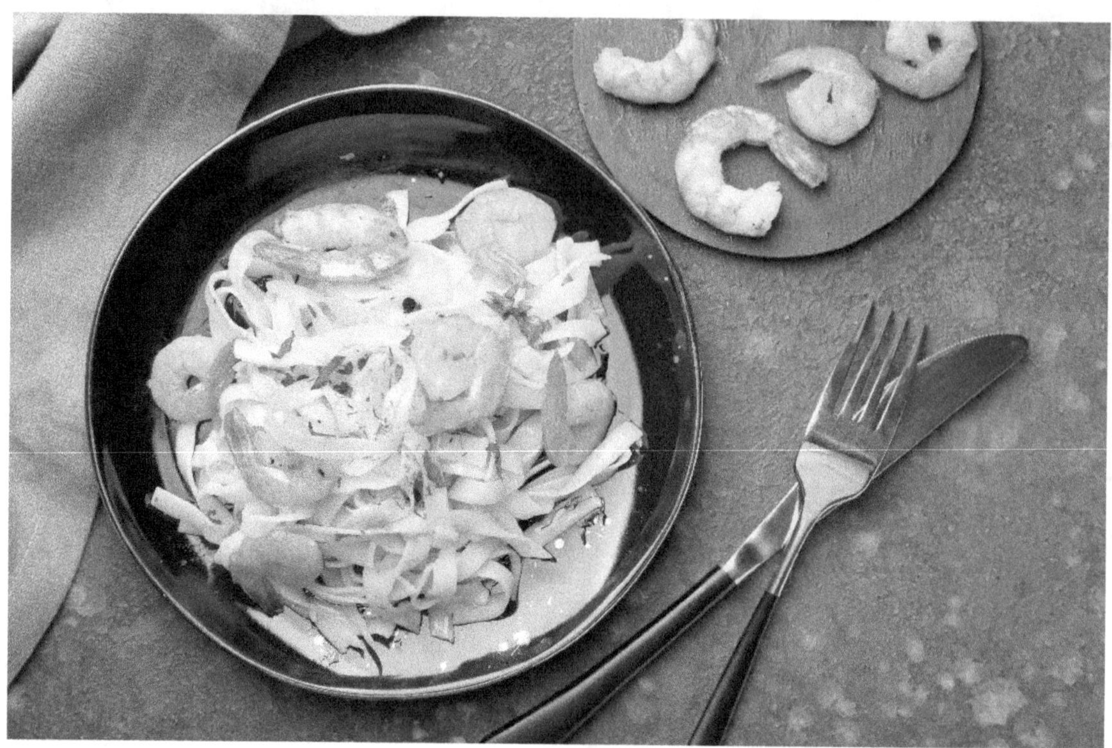

Shrimp Scampi over Whole Wheat Pasta

Preparation Time: 10 minutes | Cooking Time: 20 minutes | Portion Size: 4 servings | Difficulty Level: Easy

Ingredients:

- 12 ounces whole wheat pasta
- 1 pound shrimp, peeled and deveined
- 2 tablespoons olive oil
- 4 cloves garlic, minced
- ½ teaspoon red pepper flakes (optional)
- ½ cup low-sodium chicken broth
- ¼ cup white wine (optional)
- 2 tablespoons lemon juice
- 1 tablespoon lemon zest
- 2 tablespoons unsalted butter
- Salt and pepper to taste
- ¼ cup fresh parsley, chopped
- Lemon wedges (for serving)

Instructions:

1. **Cook the Pasta:**

    1. Bring a large pot of salted water to a boil.

    2. Add whole wheat pasta and cook according to package instructions until al dente.

    3. Drain and set aside.

2. **Prepare the Shrimp Scampi:**

    1. In a large skillet, heat olive oil over medium heat.

    2. Add garlic and red pepper flakes (if using), and sauté for 1-2 minutes until fragrant.

    3. Add shrimp and cook for 2-3 minutes on each side until pink and opaque.

4. Remove shrimp from the skillet and set aside.

3. **Make the Sauce:**

   1. In the same skillet, add chicken broth, white wine (if using), lemon juice, and lemon zest.

   2. Bring to a simmer and cook for 5 minutes until the sauce reduces slightly.

   3. Stir in butter, salt, and pepper.

4. **Combine and Serve:**

   1. Add the cooked pasta to the skillet and toss to coat in the sauce.

   2. Return the shrimp to the skillet and stir in chopped parsley.

   3. Divide the pasta and shrimp evenly among four plates.

   4. Garnish with lemon wedges and serve immediately.

Nutritional Information (per serving):

Total Carbohydrates: 45g | **Fiber:** 8g | **Sugars:** 2g | **Protein:** 28g | **Total Fat:** 12g | **Saturated Fat:** 4g | **Calories:** 360 | **Sodium:** 350mg | **Calcium:** 110mg | **Iron:** 3mg

Chicken Parmesan with Low-Fat Mozzarella

Preparation Time: 15 minutes | Cooking Time: 30 minutes | Portion Size: 4 servings | Difficulty Level: Medium

Ingredients:

Chicken:

- 4 boneless, skinless chicken breasts
- 1 cup breadcrumbs (whole wheat or gluten-free)
- ½ cup grated Parmesan cheese
- 1 teaspoon garlic powder
- 1 teaspoon onion powder
- 1 teaspoon dried oregano
- 1 teaspoon dried basil
- Salt and pepper to taste
- 2 eggs, beaten
- 1 tablespoon olive oil

Tomato Sauce:

- 2 tablespoons olive oil
- 1 small onion, diced
- 2 cloves garlic, minced
- 1 can (28 ounces) crushed tomatoes
- 1 teaspoon oregano
- 1 teaspoon basil
- 1 teaspoon thyme
- Salt and pepper to taste

Assembly:

- 1 ½ cups shredded low-fat mozzarella cheese
- ¼ cup grated Parmesan cheese
- Fresh basil leaves, chopped (for garnish)

Instructions:

1. **Prepare the Chicken:**

   1. Preheat the oven to 375°F (190°C).

   2. In a shallow bowl, mix breadcrumbs, grated Parmesan cheese, garlic powder, onion

powder, oregano, basil, salt, and pepper.

3. In another shallow bowl, beat the eggs.

4. Dip each chicken breast in the beaten eggs and then coat evenly in the breadcrumb mixture.

5. In a large skillet, heat 1 tablespoon of olive oil over medium-high heat.

6. Add the breaded chicken breasts and cook for 3-4 minutes on each side until golden brown.

7. Transfer the chicken breasts to a baking dish.

2. **Prepare the Tomato Sauce:**

1. In a medium saucepan, heat 2 tablespoons of olive oil over medium heat.

2. Add onion and garlic, and sauté for 3-4 minutes until softened.

3. Stir in crushed tomatoes, oregano, basil, thyme, salt, and pepper.

4. Bring to a simmer and cook for 15 minutes, stirring occasionally.

3. **Assemble and Bake:**

1. Spoon the tomato sauce over each chicken breast in the baking dish.

2. Sprinkle with shredded mozzarella cheese and grated Parmesan cheese.

3. Bake in the preheated oven for 15-20 minutes until the cheese is melted and bubbly.

4. **Serve:**

1. Garnish with chopped basil leaves and serve immediately.

Nutritional Information (per serving):

Total Carbohydrates: 20g | **Fiber:** 3g | **Sugars:** 5g | **Protein:** 36g | **Total Fat:** 12g | **Saturated Fat:** 4g | **Calories:** 350 | **Sodium:** 520mg | **Calcium:** 200mg | **Iron:** 3mg

Stuffed Bell Peppers with Ground Turkey and Farro

Preparation Time: 15 minutes | Cooking Time: 30 minutes | Portion Size: 4 servings | Difficulty Level: Medium

Ingredients:

- 4 large bell peppers (any color)

- 1 cup cooked farro

- 1 pound ground turkey

- 1 small onion, diced

- 2 cloves garlic, minced

- 1 zucchini, diced

- 1 can (15 ounces) diced tomatoes, drained

- 1 teaspoon cumin

- 1 teaspoon smoked paprika

- 1 teaspoon oregano

- Salt and pepper to taste

- 1 cup shredded low-fat mozzarella cheese

- ¼ cup grated Parmesan cheese

- 2 tablespoons olive oil

- Fresh parsley, chopped (for garnish)

Instructions:

1. **Prepare the Bell Peppers:**

1. Preheat the oven to 375°F (190°C).

2. Cut off the tops of the bell peppers and remove the seeds and membranes.

3. Rub the peppers with olive oil, and place them in a baking dish.

2. **Prepare the Filling:**

    1. In a large skillet, heat olive oil over medium-high heat.

    2. Add onion and garlic, and sauté for 3-4 minutes until softened.

    3. Add ground turkey and cook for 5-6 minutes until browned.

    4. Stir in zucchini, diced tomatoes, cumin, smoked paprika, oregano, salt, and pepper.

    5. Add cooked farro and mix well to combine.

    6. Cook for another 5 minutes until the mixture is heated through.

3. **Stuff the Peppers:**

    1. Spoon the turkey and farro mixture into each bell pepper, packing them tightly.

    2. Top each pepper with shredded mozzarella cheese and grated Parmesan cheese.

4. **Bake the Peppers:**

    1. Cover the baking dish with foil and bake in the preheated oven for 20 minutes.

    2. Remove the foil and bake for another 10 minutes until the cheese is melted and bubbly.

5. **Serve:**

    1. Garnish with chopped parsley and serve immediately.

Nutritional Information (per serving):

Total Carbohydrates: 35g | **Fiber:** 6g | **Sugars:** 8g | **Protein:** 28g | **Total Fat:** 12g | **Saturated Fat:** 4g | **Calories:** 350 | **Sodium:** 420mg | **Calcium:** 200mg | **Iron:** 3mg

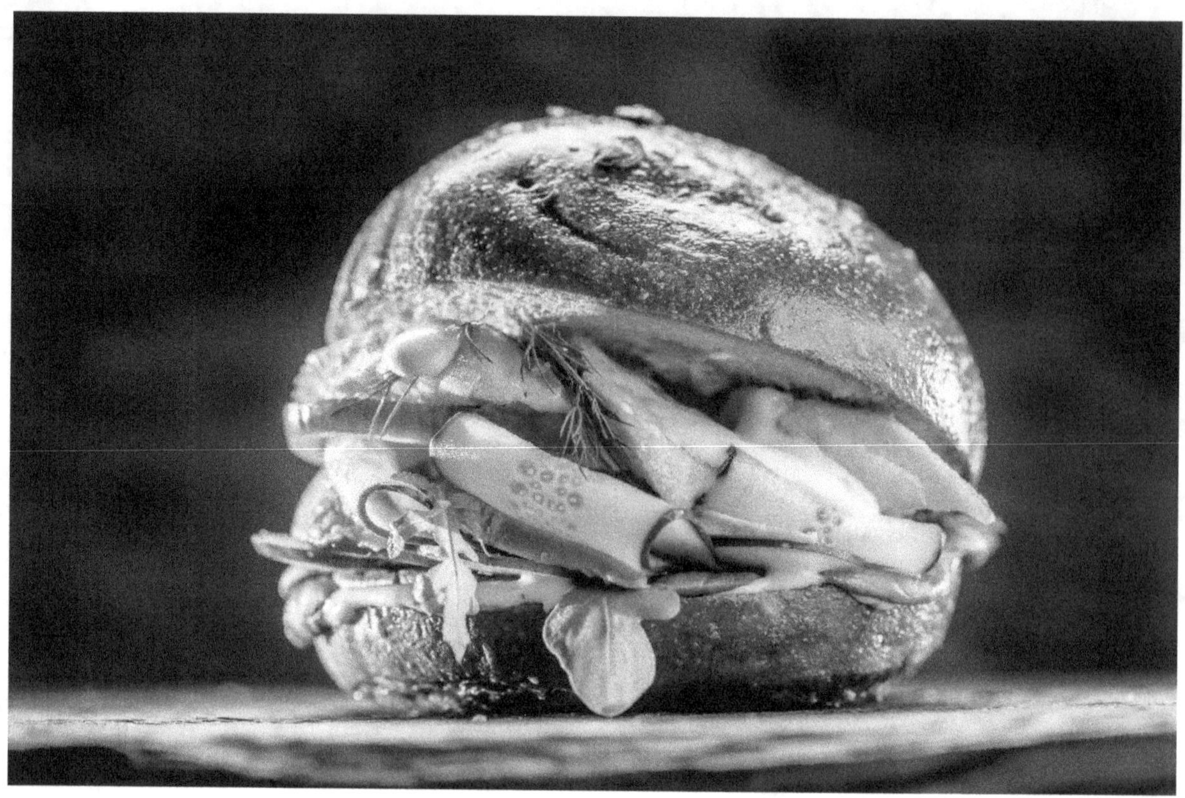

Salmon Burgers with Avocado Salsa

Preparation Time: 15 minutes | Cooking Time: 10 minutes | Portion Size: 4 servings | Difficulty Level: Medium

Ingredients:

Salmon Burgers:

- 1 ½ pounds salmon fillets, skin removed and diced
- 1 egg, beaten
- ¼ cup breadcrumbs
- 2 green onions, chopped
- 2 tablespoons fresh parsley, chopped
- 1 tablespoon Dijon mustard
- 1 tablespoon lemon juice
- 1 teaspoon smoked paprika
- 1 teaspoon garlic powder
- Salt and pepper to taste
- 1 tablespoon olive oil

Avocado Salsa:

- 1 ripe avocado, diced
- 1 small tomato, diced
- 2 tablespoons red onion, diced
- 1 tablespoon fresh cilantro, chopped
- 1 tablespoon lime juice
- Salt and pepper to taste

Assembly:

- 4 whole wheat burger buns
- 4 lettuce leaves
- Lemon wedges (for serving)

Instructions:

1. **Prepare the Salmon Burgers:**

    1. In a large bowl, combine diced salmon, beaten egg, breadcrumbs, green onions, parsley, Dijon mustard, lemon juice, smoked paprika, garlic powder, salt, and pepper.

    2. Mix well and form the mixture into four patties.

    3. In a large skillet, heat olive oil over medium-high heat.

    4. Add the salmon patties to the skillet and cook for 4-5 minutes per side until golden brown and cooked through.

2. **Prepare the Avocado Salsa:**

    1. In a medium bowl, combine diced avocado, tomato, red onion, cilantro, lime juice, salt, and pepper.

    2. Mix gently and set aside.

3. **Assemble the Burgers:**

    1. Toast the whole wheat burger buns.

    2. Place a lettuce leaf on the bottom half of each bun.

    3. Add a salmon burger patty on top of the lettuce.

    4. Spoon a generous amount of avocado salsa over the burger.

    5. Cover with the top half of the bun.

4. **Serve:**

    1. Serve immediately with lemon wedges and enjoy!

Nutritional Information (per serving):

Total Carbohydrates: 28g | **Fiber:** 7g | **Sugars:** 4g | **Protein:** 30g | **Total Fat:** 18g | **Saturated Fat:** 3.5g | **Calories:** 370 | **Sodium:** 420mg | **Calcium:** 80mg | **Iron:** 2mg

Baked Trout with Walnut Crust

Preparation Time: 10 minutes | Cooking Time: 15 minutes | Portion Size: 4 servings | Difficulty Level: Easy

Ingredients:

- 4 trout fillets (6 ounces each)
- 2 tablespoons olive oil
- 1 cup walnuts, finely chopped
- ¼ cup breadcrumbs
- 1 teaspoon thyme
- 1 teaspoon garlic powder
- ½ teaspoon smoked paprika
- Salt and pepper to taste
- Lemon wedges (for serving)

Instructions:

1. **Preheat Oven:**

    1. Preheat the oven to 400°F (200°C).

    2. Line a baking sheet with parchment paper.

2. **Prepare Walnut Crust:**

    1. In a medium bowl, combine chopped walnuts, breadcrumbs, thyme, garlic powder, smoked paprika, salt, and pepper.

    2. Mix well.

3. **Prepare Trout Fillets:**

   1. Brush the trout fillets with olive oil on both sides and season with salt and pepper.

   2. Place the trout fillets on the prepared baking sheet, skin side down.

   3. Press the walnut mixture onto the top of each fillet, coating evenly.

4. **Bake Trout:**

   1. Bake the trout fillets in the preheated oven for 12-15 minutes or until the fish is fully cooked and flakes easily with a fork.

   2. If desired, broil the fillets for the last 1-2 minutes for a golden-brown crust.

5. **Serve:**

   1. Serve the trout fillets with lemon wedges and enjoy immediately.

Nutritional Information (per serving):

Total Carbohydrates: 8g | **Fiber:** 2g | **Sugars:** 1g | **Protein:** 28g | **Total Fat:** 16g | **Saturated Fat:** 2g | **Calories:** 280 | **Sodium:** 170mg | **Calcium:** 60mg | **Iron:** 2mg

Beef and Vegetable Kabobs with Yogurt Sauce

Preparation Time: 20 minutes | Cooking Time: 10 minutes | Portion Size: 4 servings | Difficulty Level: Medium

Ingredients:

Beef and Vegetable Kabobs:

- 1 pound sirloin steak, cut into 1-inch cubes
- 1 zucchini, sliced into rounds
- 1 yellow squash, sliced into rounds
- 1 red bell pepper, cut into 1-inch pieces
- 1 yellow bell pepper, cut into 1-inch pieces
- 1 red onion, cut into 1-inch pieces
- 2 tablespoons olive oil
- 2 tablespoons lemon juice
- 2 cloves garlic, minced
- 1 teaspoon smoked paprika
- 1 teaspoon cumin
- 1 teaspoon oregano
- Salt and pepper to taste

Yogurt Sauce:

- 1 cup Greek yogurt
- 2 tablespoons lemon juice
- 2 tablespoons fresh parsley, chopped
- 1 tablespoon fresh mint, chopped
- 1 clove garlic, minced
- Salt and pepper to taste

Assembly:

- Wooden or metal skewers (if using wooden skewers, soak them in water for 30 minutes before use)

Instructions:

1. **Prepare the Marinade and Kabobs:**

   1. In a large bowl, combine olive oil, lemon juice, garlic, smoked paprika, cumin, oregano, salt, and pepper.

   2. Add the beef cubes to the bowl and toss to coat evenly.

3. Cover and marinate for at least 30 minutes.

4. Thread the marinated beef, zucchini, yellow squash, bell peppers, and red onion onto the skewers in an alternating pattern.

2. **Prepare the Yogurt Sauce:**

   1. In a small bowl, combine Greek yogurt, lemon juice, parsley, mint, garlic, salt, and pepper.

   2. Mix well and set aside.

3. **Grill the Kabobs:**

   1. Preheat the grill to medium-high heat.

   2. Grill the kabobs for 8-10 minutes, turning occasionally, until the beef is cooked to the desired doneness and the vegetables are tender.

4. **Serve:**

   1. Divide the kabobs evenly among four plates.

   2. Serve with the yogurt sauce on the side and enjoy immediately.

Nutritional Information (per serving):

Total Carbohydrates: 14g | **Fiber:** 4g | **Sugars:** 6g | **Protein:** 30g | **Total Fat:** 15g | **Saturated Fat:** 5g | **Calories:** 320 | **Sodium:** 280mg | **Calcium:** 100mg | **Iron:** 3mg

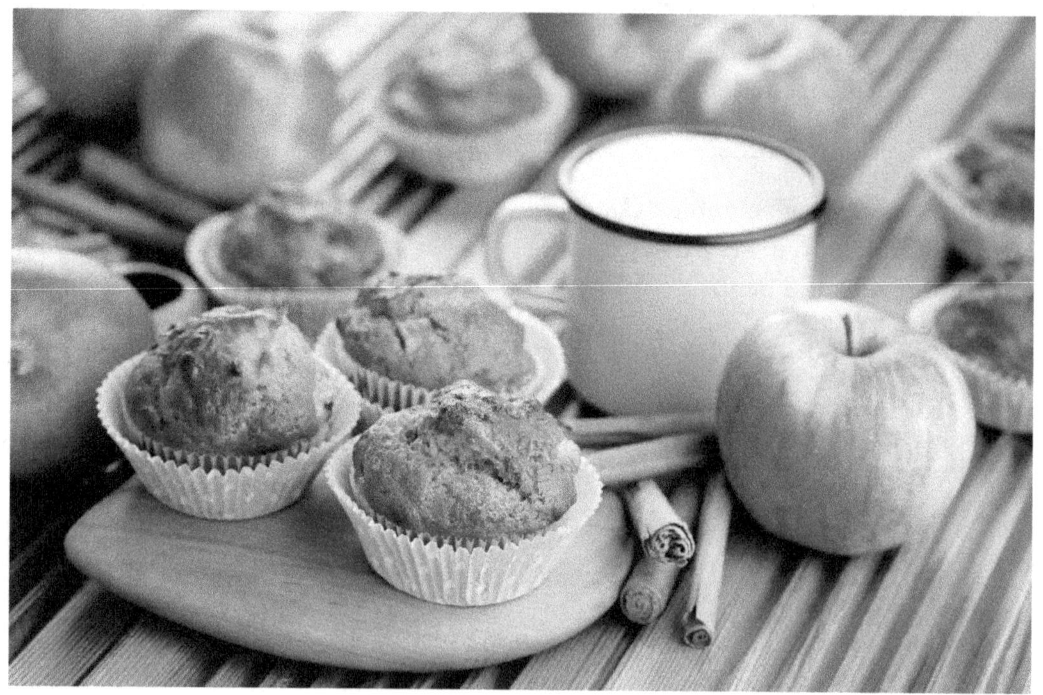

Baked Apple Cinnamon Oatmeal Cups

Preparation Time: 15 minutes | Cooking Time: 25 minutes | Portion Size: 12 cups | Difficulty Level: Easy

Ingredients:

- 2 cups rolled oats
- 1 teaspoon baking powder
- 1 teaspoon cinnamon
- ½ teaspoon nutmeg
- ½ teaspoon salt
- 1 ½ cups unsweetened almond milk
- 2 large eggs
- ¼ cup honey
- 1 teaspoon vanilla extract
- 2 apples, peeled, cored, and diced
- ¼ cup walnuts, chopped
- Cooking spray (for muffin tin)

Instructions:

1. **Preheat Oven:**

   1. Preheat the oven to 350°F (175°C).
   2. Lightly grease a 12-cup muffin tin with cooking spray or line with muffin liners.

2. **Prepare the Dry Ingredients:**

   1. In a large bowl, combine rolled oats, baking powder, cinnamon, nutmeg, and salt.
   2. Mix well.

3. **Prepare the Wet Ingredients:**

1. In a separate bowl, whisk together almond milk, eggs, honey, and vanilla extract.

4. **Combine and Add Mix-Ins:**

   1. Pour the wet ingredients into the dry ingredients and stir to combine.

   2. Fold in diced apples and chopped walnuts.

5. **Bake:**

   1. Divide the mixture evenly among the 12 muffin cups.

   2. Bake in the preheated oven for 20-25 minutes or until the oatmeal cups are set and golden brown.

   3. Let cool in the muffin tin for 5 minutes before transferring to a wire rack to cool completely.

6. **Serve:**

   1. Enjoy the baked oatmeal cups warm or at room temperature.

Nutritional Information (per serving):

Total Carbohydrates: 20g | **Fiber:** 3g | **Sugars:** 8g | **Protein:** 3g | **Total Fat:** 4g | **Saturated Fat:** 0.5g | **Calories:** 110 | **Sodium:** 120mg | **Calcium:** 40mg | **Iron:** 1mg

Low-Fat Vanilla Yogurt Parfait with Berries and Granola

Preparation Time: 10 minutes | Cooking Time: None | Portion Size: 4 servings | Difficulty Level: Easy

Ingredients:

- 2 cups low-fat vanilla Greek yogurt
- 1 cup mixed berries (e.g., strawberries, blueberries, raspberries)
- ½ cup low-fat granola
- 2 tablespoons honey
- Fresh mint leaves (for garnish)

Instructions:

1. **Prepare the Parfait Layers:**

   1. Divide ½ cup of low-fat vanilla Greek yogurt evenly among four serving glasses.

   2. Add a layer of mixed berries over the yogurt.

   3. Add a spoonful of low-fat granola on top of the berries.

   4. Repeat the layers with the remaining yogurt, berries, and granola.

2. **Finish with Honey:**

   1. Drizzle the parfaits with honey.

3. **Serve:**

   1. Garnish with fresh mint leaves.

   2. Enjoy immediately or refrigerate until ready to serve.

Nutritional Information (per serving):

Total Carbohydrates: 30g | **Fiber:** 4g | **Sugars:** 15g | **Protein:** 10g | **Total Fat:** 5g | **Saturated Fat:** 1g | **Calories:** 190 | **Sodium:** 80mg | **Calcium:** 120mg | **Iron:** 1.5mg

Carrot Cake with Low-Fat Cream Cheese Frosting

Preparation Time: 20 minutes | Cooking Time: 30 minutes | Portion Size: 12 servings | Difficulty Level: Medium

Ingredients:

Carrot Cake:

- 2 cups whole wheat flour
- 1 teaspoon baking powder
- 1 teaspoon baking soda
- 1 teaspoon cinnamon
- ½ teaspoon nutmeg
- ½ teaspoon ginger
- ½ teaspoon salt
- 3 large eggs
- ½ cup unsweetened applesauce
- ½ cup honey
- ¼ cup olive oil
- 1 teaspoon vanilla extract
- 2 cups grated carrots
- ½ cup walnuts, chopped
- ½ cup raisins (optional)

Low-Fat Cream Cheese Frosting:

- 1 (8-ounce) package low-fat cream cheese, softened
- ¼ cup powdered sugar
- 1 teaspoon vanilla extract
- 1 tablespoon unsweetened almond milk (if needed for consistency)

Instructions:

1. **Prepare the Carrot Cake:**

    1. Preheat the oven to 350°F (175°C).

    2. Grease and flour a 9x13 inch baking pan or two 8-inch round cake pans.

    3. In a medium bowl, whisk together whole wheat flour, baking powder, baking soda, cinnamon, nutmeg, ginger, and salt.

    4. In a large bowl, beat the eggs with applesauce, honey, olive oil, and vanilla extract until well combined.

    5. Gradually add the dry ingredients to the wet ingredients and mix until just combined.

    6. Fold in grated carrots, chopped walnuts, and raisins (if using).

    7. Pour the batter into the prepared pan(s) and bake for 25-30 minutes, or until a toothpick inserted into the center comes out clean.

    8. Let the cake cool completely before frosting.

2. **Prepare the Low-Fat Cream Cheese Frosting:**

    1. In a medium bowl, beat the softened cream cheese until smooth.

    2. Add powdered sugar and vanilla extract, and beat until well combined.

    3. If the frosting is too thick, add a tablespoon of unsweetened almond milk to achieve the desired consistency.

3. **Frost the Cake:**

    1. Spread the low-fat cream cheese frosting evenly over the cooled carrot cake.

2. If using two layers, frost the top of one layer, place the second layer on top, and then frost the entire cake.

4. **Serve:**

1. Slice and enjoy immediately or refrigerate until ready to serve.

Nutritional Information (per serving):

Total Carbohydrates: 28g | **Fiber:** 4g | **Sugars:** 12g | **Protein:** 6g | **Total Fat:** 10g | **Saturated Fat:** 2.5g | **Calories:** 210 | **Sodium:** 180mg | **Calcium:** 70mg | **Iron:** 2mg

Banana Nut Muffins with Whole Wheat

Preparation Time: 15 minutes | Cooking Time: 20 minutes | Portion Size: 12 muffins | Difficulty Level: Easy

Ingredients:

- 1 ½ cups whole wheat flour
- 1 teaspoon baking soda
- 1 teaspoon baking powder
- ½ teaspoon salt
- 1 teaspoon cinnamon
- 3 ripe bananas, mashed
- ½ cup honey
- ¼ cup unsweetened applesauce
- ¼ cup Greek yogurt
- 2 large eggs
- 1 teaspoon vanilla extract
- ½ cup walnuts, chopped
- ¼ cup rolled oats (for topping)

Instructions:

1. **Preheat Oven:**

   1. Preheat the oven to 350°F (175°C).

   2. Line a 12-cup muffin tin with paper liners or lightly grease with cooking spray.

2. **Prepare the Dry Ingredients:**

   1. In a medium bowl, combine whole wheat flour, baking soda, baking powder, salt, and cinnamon.

   2. Mix well and set aside.

3. **Prepare the Wet Ingredients:**

   1. In a large bowl, whisk together mashed bananas, honey, applesauce, Greek yogurt, eggs, and vanilla extract until well combined.

4. **Combine the Mixtures:**

   1. Add the dry ingredients to the wet ingredients and mix until just combined.

   2. Fold in chopped walnuts.

5. **Fill the Muffin Tin:**

   1. Divide the batter evenly among the muffin cups.

   2. Sprinkle rolled oats over the tops of the muffins.

6. **Bake:**

1. Bake in the preheated oven for 18-20 minutes, or until a toothpick inserted into the center comes out clean.

2. Let the muffins cool in the tin for 5 minutes before transferring to a wire rack to cool completely.

7. **Serve:**

1. Enjoy the muffins warm or at room temperature.

Nutritional Information (per serving):

Total Carbohydrates: 28g | **Fiber:** 4g | **Sugars:** 12g | **Protein:** 4g | **Total Fat:** 5g | **Saturated Fat:** 0.5g | **Calories:** 150 | **Sodium:** 180mg | **Calcium:** 40mg | **Iron:** 1mg

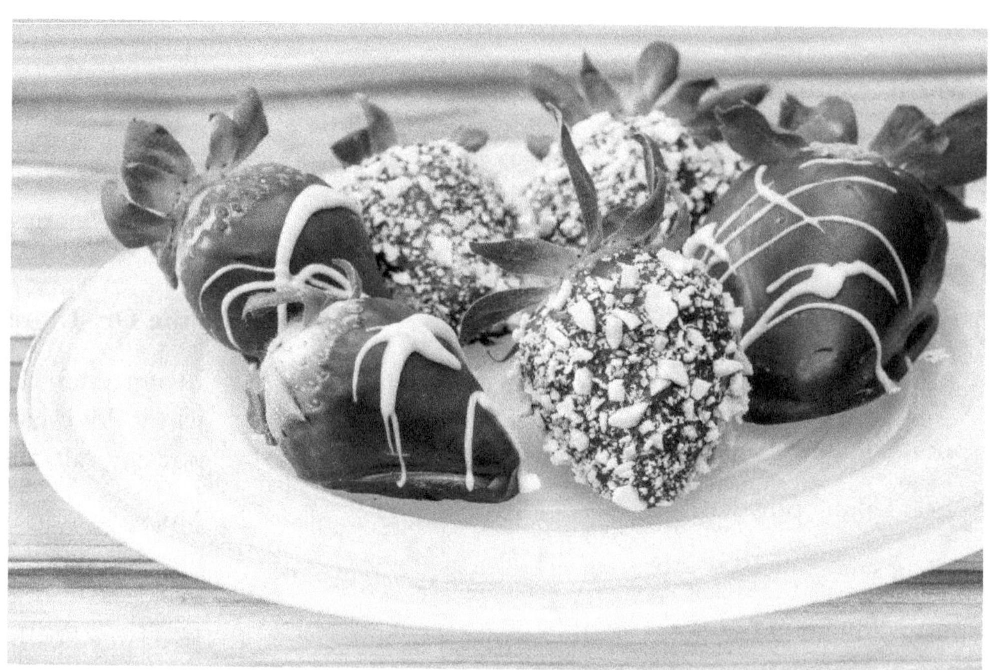

Chocolate-Dipped Strawberries with Dark Chocolate

Preparation Time: 10 minutes | Cooking Time: 5 minutes | Portion Size: 4 servings | Difficulty Level: Easy

Ingredients:

- 16 large strawberries, washed and dried

- 6 ounces dark chocolate (70% cacao or higher), chopped

- 1 teaspoon coconut oil (optional)

- 1 tablespoon chopped nuts (optional, for garnish)

- 1 tablespoon shredded coconut (optional, for garnish)

Instructions:

1. **Prepare the Chocolate:**

   1. In a heatproof bowl, combine chopped dark chocolate and coconut oil (if using).

   2. Place the bowl over a pot of simmering water (double boiler method), making sure the bottom of the bowl doesn't touch the water.

   3. Stir until the chocolate is completely melted and smooth.

4. Remove from heat and let cool slightly.

2. **Dip the Strawberries:**

    1. Line a baking sheet with parchment paper.

    2. Hold each strawberry by the stem and dip it into the melted chocolate, swirling to coat evenly.

    3. Lift the strawberry and let the excess chocolate drip off.

    4. Place the chocolate-dipped strawberry on the parchment-lined baking sheet.

    5. Repeat with the remaining strawberries.

3. **Add Garnishes (Optional):**

    1. Sprinkle chopped nuts or shredded coconut over the chocolate-dipped strawberries if desired.

4. **Chill and Serve:**

    1. Place the baking sheet in the refrigerator for 15-20 minutes, or until the chocolate is set.

    2. Serve the chocolate-dipped strawberries immediately or store them in an airtight container in the refrigerator.

Nutritional Information (per serving):

Total Carbohydrates: 18g | **Fiber:** 4g | **Sugars:** 12g | **Protein:** 2g | **Total Fat:** 10g | **Saturated Fat:** 6g | **Calories:** 150 | **Sodium:** 10mg | **Calcium:** 20mg | **Iron:** 2mg

Almond and Date Energy Balls

Preparation Time: 10 minutes | Cooking Time: None | Portion Size: 15 balls | Difficulty Level: Easy

Ingredients:

- 1 cup raw almonds
- 1 cup pitted Medjool dates
- 2 tablespoons almond butter
- 1 teaspoon vanilla extract
- ½ teaspoon cinnamon
- Pinch of salt
- 1 tablespoon chia seeds (optional)
- 1 tablespoon unsweetened shredded coconut (optional, for rolling)

Instructions:

1. **Prepare the Mixture:**

    1. In a food processor, pulse the almonds until coarsely ground.

    2. Add the dates, almond butter, vanilla extract, cinnamon, salt, and chia seeds (if using).

    3. Process until the mixture forms a sticky dough.

2. **Shape the Balls:**

    1. Scoop out about a tablespoon of the mixture and roll it into a ball using your hands.

    2. Repeat with the remaining mixture to form 15 energy balls.

    3. If desired, roll the energy balls in unsweetened shredded coconut for a coating.

3. **Chill and Serve:**

1. Place the energy balls in an airtight container and refrigerate for at least 30 minutes before serving.

2. Enjoy as a quick and healthy snack!

Coconut Water Fruit Popsicles

Preparation Time: 10 minutes | Freezing Time: 4 hours | Portion Size: 8 popsicles | Difficulty Level: Easy

Ingredients:

- 2 cups coconut water
- 1 kiwi, peeled and sliced
- 1 cup strawberries, hulled and sliced
- 1 cup blueberries
- 1 cup mango, diced
- 1 tablespoon honey (optional)

Instructions:

1. **Prepare the Fruit:**
   1. Arrange the kiwi, strawberries, blueberries, and mango evenly in the popsicle molds.

2. **Prepare the Liquid:**
   1. In a bowl, combine coconut water and honey (if using).
   2. Stir well to dissolve the honey.

3. **Fill the Molds:**
   1. Pour the coconut water mixture into each popsicle mold, covering the fruit.
   2. Insert popsicle sticks into the molds.

4. **Freeze:**
   1. Place the molds in the freezer and freeze for at least 4 hours, or until fully frozen.

5. **Serve:**
   1. Run warm water over the outside of the molds to release the popsicles.
   2. Enjoy immediately or store in the freezer until ready to serve.

Nutritional Information (per serving):

Total Carbohydrates: 10g | **Fiber:** 2g | **Sugars:** 7g | **Protein:** 0.5g | **Total Fat:** 0.2g | **Saturated Fat:** 0g | **Calories:** 40 | **Sodium:** 20mg | **Calcium:** 10mg | **Iron:** 0.3mg

Poached Pears with Cinnamon and Clove

Preparation Time: 10 minutes | Cooking Time: 25 minutes | Portion Size: 4 servings | Difficulty Level: Easy

Ingredients:

- 4 ripe but firm pears, peeled and cored
- 4 cups water
- ½ cup honey
- 1 cinnamon stick
- 3 whole cloves

Nutritional Information (per serving):

Total Carbohydrates: 12g | **Fiber:** 3g | **Sugars:** 8g | **Protein:** 3g | **Total Fat:** 5g | **Saturated Fat:** 0.5g | **Calories:** 90 | **Sodium:** 20mg | **Calcium:** 30mg | **Iron:** 0.8mg

- 1 teaspoon vanilla extract
- ½ teaspoon lemon zest
- 1 tablespoon lemon juice
- Fresh mint leaves (for garnish)

Instructions:

1. **Prepare the Poaching Liquid:**
   1. In a large pot, combine water, honey, cinnamon stick, cloves, vanilla extract, lemon zest, and lemon juice.
   2. Bring to a simmer over medium heat.

2. **Poach the Pears:**
   1. Add the peeled and cored pears to the pot.
   2. Reduce heat to low and simmer gently for 20-25 minutes, turning occasionally until the pears are tender but not mushy.
   3. Carefully remove the pears from the poaching liquid and set aside.

3. **Reduce the Poaching Liquid:**
   1. Increase heat to medium-high and simmer the poaching liquid for an additional 10 minutes until slightly reduced and syrupy.

4. **Serve:**
   1. Place the poached pears on serving plates.
   2. Drizzle with the reduced poaching liquid and garnish with fresh mint leaves.
   3. Serve warm or chilled.

Nutritional Information (per serving):

Total Carbohydrates: 35g | **Fiber:** 5g | **Sugars:** 30g | **Protein:** 1g | **Total Fat:** 0.2g | **Saturated Fat:** 0g | **Calories:** 140 | **Sodium:** 10mg | **Calcium:** 10mg | **Iron:** 0.3mg

Raspberry Chia Seed Pudding

Preparation Time: 10 minutes | Chilling Time: 4 hours | Portion Size: 4 servings | Difficulty Level: Easy

Ingredients:

- 1 ½ cups unsweetened almond milk
- ½ cup chia seeds
- 2 tablespoons honey or maple syrup
- 1 teaspoon vanilla extract
- 1 cup fresh or frozen raspberries
- Fresh mint leaves (for garnish)

Instructions:

1. **Prepare the Pudding Base:**
   1. In a medium bowl, whisk together unsweetened almond milk, chia seeds, honey or maple syrup, and vanilla extract.
   2. Stir in raspberries, lightly crushing them with a spoon to release their juices.
   3. Cover and refrigerate for at least 4 hours or overnight until the pudding thickens.

2. **Serve:**
   1. Divide the raspberry chia seed pudding evenly among four serving bowls.
   2. Garnish with fresh mint leaves.

3. Enjoy immediately or store in the refrigerator until ready to serve.

Nutritional Information (per serving):

Total Carbohydrates: 14g | **Fiber:** 8g | **Sugars:** 6g | **Protein:** 4g | **Total Fat:** 8g | **Saturated Fat:** 1g | **Calories:** 140 | **Sodium:** 30mg | **Calcium:** 150mg | **Iron:** 2mg

Baked Peaches with Honey and Almonds

Preparation Time: 10 minutes | Cooking Time: 15 minutes | Portion Size: 4 servings | Difficulty Level: Easy

Ingredients:

- 4 ripe peaches, halved and pitted
- 2 tablespoons honey
- ¼ cup sliced almonds
- ½ teaspoon cinnamon
- 1 teaspoon vanilla extract
- 1 tablespoon unsweetened almond milk
- Fresh mint leaves (for garnish)

Instructions:

1. **Preheat Oven:**
   1. Preheat the oven to 375°F (190°C).
   2. Line a baking sheet with parchment paper.
2. **Prepare the Peaches:**
   1. Place the peach halves cut side up on the prepared baking sheet.
3. **Prepare the Honey-Almond Topping:**
   1. In a small bowl, combine honey, sliced almonds, cinnamon, vanilla extract, and almond milk.
   2. Mix well.
4. **Bake:**
   1. Spoon the honey-almond mixture evenly over each peach half.
   2. Bake in the preheated oven for 12-15 minutes until the peaches are tender and the topping is golden.
5. **Serve:**
   1. Garnish the baked peaches with fresh mint leaves.
   2. Enjoy immediately or serve with Greek yogurt or whipped cream if desired.

Nutritional Information (per serving):

Total Carbohydrates: 16g | **Fiber:** 3g | **Sugars:** 13g | **Protein:** 2g | **Total Fat:** 4g | **Saturated Fat:** 0.5g | **Calories:** 110 | **Sodium:** 5mg | **Calcium:** 20mg | **Iron:** 0.8mg

Mango and Sticky Rice

Preparation Time: 15 minutes | Cooking Time: 30 minutes | Portion Size: 4 servings | Difficulty Level: Medium

Ingredients:

Sticky Rice:

- 1 cup glutinous (sticky) rice
- 1 ½ cups coconut milk
- ½ cup water
- ¼ cup sugar

- ¼ teaspoon salt

Mango Topping:

- 2 ripe mangoes, peeled, pitted, and sliced

Coconut Sauce:

- ½ cup coconut milk
- 2 tablespoons sugar
- ¼ teaspoon salt
- 1 teaspoon cornstarch
- 2 teaspoons water

Instructions:

1. **Prepare the Sticky Rice:**

   1. Rinse the sticky rice under cold water until the water runs clear.
   2. Soak the rice in water for at least 4 hours or overnight.
   3. Drain the rice and transfer it to a steamer lined with cheesecloth or a banana leaf.
   4. Steam the rice over boiling water for 20-25 minutes until tender.

2. **Prepare the Coconut Sauce:**

   1. In a small saucepan, combine coconut milk, sugar, and salt.
   2. Heat over medium heat, stirring frequently until the sugar dissolves. Do not boil.
   3. In a small bowl, mix cornstarch with water to create a slurry.
   4. Stir the slurry into the coconut milk mixture and continue to cook until slightly thickened.

3. **Combine the Sticky Rice with Coconut Sauce:**

   1. Transfer the cooked sticky rice to a mixing bowl.
   2. Pour 1 cup of the warm coconut sauce over the rice and mix gently.
   3. Let the rice sit for 10 minutes to absorb the coconut sauce.

4. **Serve:**

   1. Divide the sticky rice among four plates.
   2. Arrange the sliced mangoes on top or on the side of the sticky rice.
   3. Drizzle additional coconut sauce over the rice and mangoes.
   4. Enjoy immediately.

Nutritional Information (per serving):

Total Carbohydrates: 55g | **Fiber:** 3g | **Sugars:** 18g | **Protein:** 3g | **Total Fat:** 9g | **Saturated Fat:** 8g | **Calories:** 320 | **Sodium:** 120mg | **Calcium:** 30mg | **Iron:** 1mg

Blueberry Lemon Zest Muffins

Preparation Time: 15 minutes | Cooking Time: 20 minutes | Portion Size: 12 muffins | Difficulty Level: Easy

Ingredients:

- 1 ½ cups whole wheat flour
- ½ cup rolled oats
- 1 teaspoon baking powder
- 1 teaspoon baking soda
- ½ teaspoon salt

- 1 teaspoon cinnamon
- 2 large eggs
- ½ cup honey
- ¼ cup Greek yogurt
- ¼ cup unsweetened applesauce
- 2 tablespoons olive oil
- 1 teaspoon vanilla extract
- 1 tablespoon lemon zest
- 1 cup blueberries (fresh or frozen)
- 2 tablespoons rolled oats (for topping)

Instructions:

1. **Preheat Oven:**
   1. Preheat the oven to 375°F (190°C).
   2. Line a 12-cup muffin tin with paper liners or lightly grease with cooking spray.

2. **Prepare the Dry Ingredients:**
   1. In a medium bowl, combine whole wheat flour, rolled oats, baking powder, baking soda, salt, and cinnamon.
   2. Mix well and set aside.

3. **Prepare the Wet Ingredients:**
   1. In a large bowl, whisk together eggs, honey, Greek yogurt, applesauce, olive oil, vanilla extract, and lemon zest.

4. **Combine the Mixtures:**
   1. Add the dry ingredients to the wet ingredients and mix until just combined.
   2. Gently fold in the blueberries.

5. **Fill the Muffin Tin:**
   1. Divide the batter evenly among the muffin cups.
   2. Sprinkle rolled oats over the tops of the muffins.

6. **Bake:**
   1. Bake in the preheated oven for 18-20 minutes, or until a toothpick inserted into the center comes out clean.
   2. Let the muffins cool in the tin for 5 minutes before transferring to a wire rack to cool completely.

7. **Serve:**
   1. Enjoy the muffins warm or at room temperature.

Nutritional Information (per serving):

Total Carbohydrates: 26g | **Fiber:** 4g | **Sugars:** 10g | **Protein:** 4g | **Total Fat:** 5g | **Saturated Fat:** 0.5g | **Calories:** 150 | **Sodium:** 180mg | **Calcium:** 40mg | **Iron:** 1mg

Apple and Walnut Crisp with Oat Topping

Preparation Time: 15 minutes | Cooking Time: 35 minutes | Portion Size: 8 servings | Difficulty Level: Easy

Ingredients:

Filling:

- 6 cups apples, peeled, cored, and sliced
- ¼ cup honey
- 1 tablespoon lemon juice
- 1 teaspoon cinnamon

- ¼ teaspoon nutmeg
- ¼ teaspoon salt

Oat Topping:

- 1 cup rolled oats
- ½ cup whole wheat flour
- ½ cup walnuts, chopped
- ⅓ cup coconut oil, melted
- ⅓ cup honey
- 1 teaspoon cinnamon
- ¼ teaspoon salt

Instructions:

1. **Preheat Oven:**
    1. Preheat the oven to 350°F (175°C).
    2. Grease a 9x13 inch baking dish with cooking spray.

2. **Prepare the Filling:**
    1. In a large bowl, combine apples, honey, lemon juice, cinnamon, nutmeg, and salt.
    2. Mix well and transfer the mixture to the prepared baking dish.

3. **Prepare the Oat Topping:**
    1. In a medium bowl, combine rolled oats, whole wheat flour, chopped walnuts, coconut oil, honey, cinnamon, and salt.
    2. Mix well until the topping resembles coarse crumbs.

4. **Assemble and Bake:**
    1. Sprinkle the oat topping evenly over the apple mixture.
    2. Bake in the preheated oven for 30-35 minutes, or until the topping is golden brown and the apples are tender.

5. **Serve:**
    1. Let the apple and walnut crisp cool for 10 minutes before serving.
    2. Enjoy warm or at room temperature.

Nutritional Information (per serving):

Total Carbohydrates: 42g | **Fiber:** 6g | **Sugars:** 22g | **Protein:** 4g | **Total Fat:** 9g | **Saturated Fat:** 4g | **Calories:** 220 | **Sodium:** 100mg | **Calcium:** 40mg | **Iron:** 1.5mg

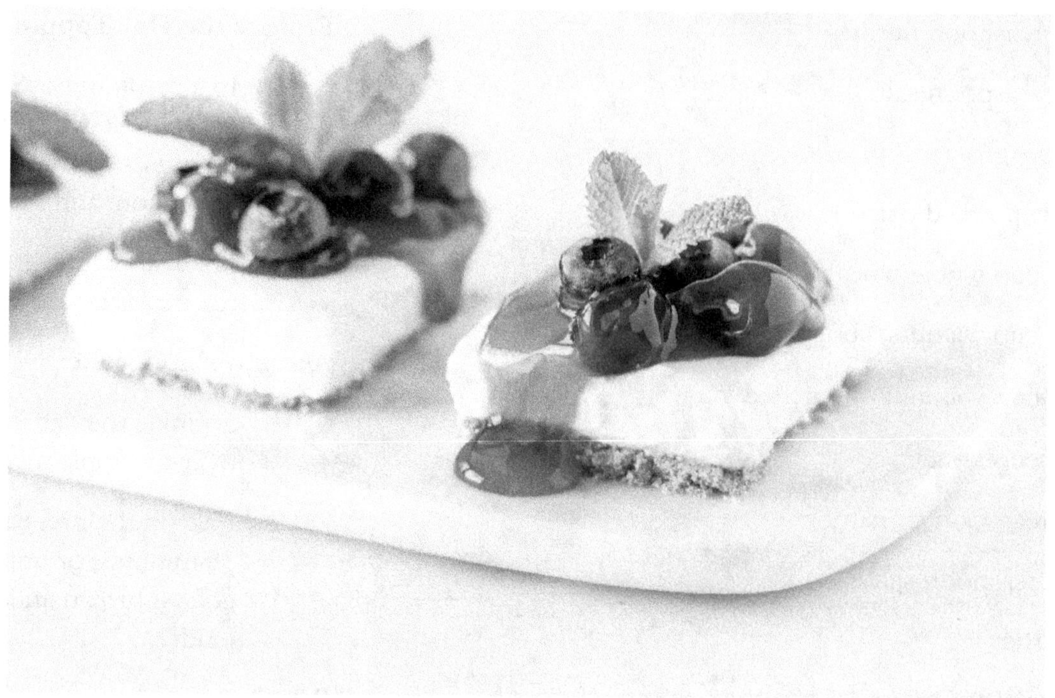

Low-Fat Cheesecake with Fresh Fruit Topping

Preparation Time: 20 minutes | Cooking Time: 50 minutes | Chilling Time: 4 hours | Portion Size: 8 servings | Difficulty Level: Medium

Ingredients:

Crust:

- 1 cup graham cracker crumbs
- 2 tablespoons sugar
- 2 tablespoons melted coconut oil

Filling:

- 16 ounces low-fat cream cheese, softened
- ½ cup Greek yogurt
- ½ cup honey
- 2 large eggs
- 2 teaspoons vanilla extract
- 1 tablespoon lemon juice
- 1 teaspoon lemon zest

Fruit Topping:

- 1 cup mixed berries (e.g., strawberries, blueberries, raspberries)
- 2 tablespoons honey
- 1 tablespoon lemon juice

Instructions:

1. **Preheat Oven:**

   1. Preheat the oven to 325°F (160°C).
   2. Grease a 9-inch springform pan.

2. **Prepare the Crust:**

   1. In a medium bowl, mix graham cracker crumbs, sugar, and melted coconut oil.
   2. Press the mixture firmly into the bottom of the prepared springform pan.
   3. Bake for 8-10 minutes until lightly golden.

4. Remove from the oven and set aside.

3. **Prepare the Filling:**

   1. In a large bowl, beat together softened cream cheese, Greek yogurt, and honey until smooth.

   2. Add eggs one at a time, mixing well after each addition.

   3. Stir in vanilla extract, lemon juice, and lemon zest.

   4. Pour the filling over the prepared crust.

4. **Bake the Cheesecake:**

   1. Bake in the preheated oven for 45-50 minutes until the edges are set and the center is slightly jiggly.

   2. Turn off the oven, crack the door open, and let the cheesecake cool in the oven for 1 hour.

   3. Transfer to the refrigerator and chill for at least 4 hours or overnight.

5. **Prepare the Fruit Topping:**

   1. In a medium bowl, mix mixed berries, honey, and lemon juice.

   2. Let the mixture sit for 10 minutes to macerate.

6. **Serve:**

   1. Run a knife around the edge of the cheesecake to loosen it from the pan.

   2. Remove the sides of the springform pan.

   3. Spoon the fruit topping over the cheesecake.

   4. Slice and enjoy!

Nutritional Information (per serving):

Total Carbohydrates: 28g | **Fiber:** 2g | **Sugars:** 22g | **Protein:** 8g | **Total Fat:** 8g | **Saturated Fat:** 4g | **Calories:** 210 | **Sodium:** 180mg | **Calcium:** 70mg | **Iron:** 1mg

No-Bake Peanut Butter Cookies

Preparation Time: 10 minutes | Chilling Time: 30 minutes | Portion Size: 12 cookies | Difficulty Level: Easy

Ingredients:

- 1 cup rolled oats
- ½ cup natural peanut butter
- ¼ cup honey
- ¼ cup unsweetened shredded coconut
- 1 teaspoon vanilla extract
- ¼ teaspoon salt
- 2 tablespoons chia seeds (optional)
- 2 tablespoons mini chocolate chips (optional)

Instructions:

1. **Prepare the Mixture:**

   1. In a large bowl, mix rolled oats, peanut butter, honey, shredded coconut, vanilla extract, salt, chia seeds (if using), and mini chocolate chips (if using).

   2. Stir until well combined.

2. **Shape the Cookies:**

1. Scoop out about a tablespoon of the mixture and roll it into a ball using your hands.

2. Flatten the ball to form a cookie shape.

3. Repeat with the remaining mixture to form 12 cookies.

3. **Chill and Serve:**

   1. Place the cookies on a parchment-lined baking sheet.

   2. Refrigerate for at least 30 minutes or until firm.

   3. Enjoy immediately or store in an airtight container in the refrigerator.

Nutritional Information (per serving):

Total Carbohydrates: 15g | **Fiber:** 3g | **Sugars:** 7g | **Protein:** 4g | **Total Fat:** 8g | **Saturated Fat:** 2g | **Calories:** 130 | **Sodium:** 80mg | **Calcium:** 20mg | **Iron:** 0.8mg

Part III: Comfort Digest Formula

Foundation of Comfort Digest: Understanding Your New Digestive Dynamics

Adjusting to life without a gallbladder involves a deep understanding of how your digestive system now functions, particularly concerning bile production and its role in digestion. Here's what you need to know to adapt and maintain digestive comfort.

The Role of Bile in Digestion

Bile, a critical digestive fluid produced by the liver, aids in the digestion and absorption of fats. In a gallbladder-bearing digestive system, bile is stored in the gallbladder and released in significant amounts when you consume fat. This targeted release helps efficiently break down and absorb dietary fats.

Changes After Gallbladder Removal

After gallbladder removal, also known as a cholecystectomy, the bile is no longer stored but drips continuously into the small intestine. This change presents two main challenges:

1. **Continuous Drip vs. Concentrated Release:** Without the gallbladder's capacity to release bile in response to fatty meals, the continuous drip can be insufficient to handle large amounts of fat at one time. This can lead to incomplete digestion of fats, which may cause digestive discomforts such as bloating, gas, and diarrhea.

2. **Increased Risk of Bile Acidity:** The constant presence of bile in the intestine, regardless of food intake, can lead to an increased risk of developing bile acid diarrhea. Additionally, the altered flow of bile may also contribute to the development of small intestine bacterial overgrowth (SIBO), as the antibacterial action of concentrated bile releases is diminished.

Adapting Your Diet

To accommodate these changes, dietary adaptations are necessary:

- **Moderate Fat Consumption:** Since large amounts of fats can overwhelm your new digestive system, it's advisable to moderate your fat intake. This doesn't mean all fats need to be avoided—rather, the focus should be on consuming easily digestible, healthier fats in controlled portions throughout the day.

- **Frequent, Smaller Meals:** Eating smaller, more frequent meals can prevent the overload of bile and help maintain a smoother digestion process. This eating pattern allows bile to be utilized more effectively as it continues to flow into the intestine.

- **Incorporate Soluble Fiber:** Soluble fiber can bind to bile acids, potentially reducing symptoms of bile acid diarrhea. Foods rich in soluble fiber include oats, apples, carrots, and beans, which can also help regulate digestion and support overall intestinal health.

Monitoring and Adjusting

Understanding and monitoring how your body reacts to different foods and adjusting your diet accordingly are crucial. Keeping a detailed food diary, as discussed in earlier sections, can help you pinpoint which foods exacerbate symptoms and which support your digestive health. This ongoing personal feedback loop will be instrumental in shaping a diet that not only minimizes discomfort but also enhances your quality of life.

This foundational knowledge of your new digestive dynamics underpins the entire Comfort Digest Formula, equipping you with the insights needed to navigate this transition effectively. By embracing these changes and adapting your lifestyle, you can achieve a balanced and comfortable digestive state.

Nutritional Building Blocks: Customized Nutrient Management

As you adapt to life without a gallbladder, understanding the nutritional building blocks—macronutrients and micronutrients—becomes essential for maintaining balance and comfort. This section will guide you through the crucial aspects of customizing your nutrient intake to support your altered digestive system effectively.

Managing Macronutrients

1. **Proteins:** Proteins are vital for tissue repair and growth. They do not significantly stimulate bile release, making them a safe choice for a gallbladder-free diet. Focus on lean sources of protein such as chicken, fish, turkey, and plant-based proteins like lentils and tofu to ensure you receive adequate nutrition without overloading your digestive system.

2. **Carbohydrates:** Carbohydrates should be consumed primarily in the form of whole grains, fruits, and vegetables, which provide energy as well as essential fibers. These fibers help regulate the digestive system and can bind to bile acids, reducing potential irritation. Avoid simple sugars and refined carbs, which can cause rapid bile secretion spikes that your body may not handle well.

3. **Fats:** Even without a gallbladder, fats remain an essential part of your diet. However, the key is to choose fats that are easier to digest. Incorporate moderate amounts of healthy fats like those found in avocados, nuts, seeds, and olive oil throughout the day. This helps ensure that the continuous drip of bile has a regular use, reducing the chances of digestive discomfort.

Importance of Micronutrients

Managing micronutrients is equally important, particularly fat-soluble vitamins (A, D, E, and K), which may be harder to absorb due to changes in bile availability. Here's how to ensure you're getting enough:

- **Vitamin A:** Necessary for skin health and vision. Include carrots, sweet potatoes, and leafy greens in your diet.

- **Vitamin D:** Essential for bone health and immune function. Besides sunlight exposure, consider fortified foods or supplements as per your doctor's advice.

- **Vitamin E:** Important for protecting body tissue from damage and supporting immune health. Nuts and seeds are good sources.

- **Vitamin K:** Plays a critical role in blood clotting and bone health. Leafy greens like spinach and kale are rich in vitamin K.

Supplement Considerations

Due to altered fat digestion, you might need supplements to ensure adequate intake of certain nutrients. Consult with a healthcare provider to determine if you need supplements based on your specific health profile and dietary intake. This could include multivitamins or specific supplements like omega-3 fatty acids, which are beneficial for overall health and may be difficult to absorb sufficiently from diet alone.

Customizing Your Diet

Every individual's body reacts differently post-gallbladder removal. It's crucial to listen to your body and adjust your diet according to how you respond to different foods. Utilizing the insights gained from a food diary (as recommended in the Daily Digest Tracker) will help you fine-tune your nutritional intake, ensuring that your diet not only meets your nutritional needs but also supports your digestion and overall well-being.

By understanding and managing these nutritional building blocks, you can create a supportive dietary environment that enhances your life without a gallbladder. This approach not only minimizes discomfort but also ensures that your body receives the nutrients it needs to function optimally.

Bloat-Busting Recipe Design: Creating the Perfect Meal

Designing meals that minimize bloating and maximize comfort is crucial for those living without a gallbladder. A focus on low-fat, high-fiber ingredients forms the foundation of bloat-busting recipes, helping to manage digestion and maintain satisfaction. This section outlines the principles of crafting meals that support your digestive system without triggering discomfort.

Low-Fat Cooking Techniques

Since excessive fat can be hard to digest without a gallbladder, utilizing low-fat cooking techniques is essential:

- **Grilling, Baking, and Broiling:** These methods allow you to cook foods thoroughly without adding extra fat.

- **Steaming:** Cooking vegetables, fish, and even some cuts of poultry by steaming preserves nutrients and does not require fat.

- **Using Broths:** Instead of frying with oils, try sautéing with vegetable or chicken broth to add flavor without the fat.

High-Fiber Content

Incorporating a high fiber content in your meals helps regulate digestion and can bind to excess bile acids:

- **Whole Grains:** Opt for whole grains like quinoa, brown rice, and whole-wheat pasta which provide a good source of fiber.

- **Legumes:** Beans, lentils, and chickpeas are excellent high-fiber additions to any meal.

- **Vegetables and Fruits:** Aim to include a variety of vegetables and fruits in your meals, focusing on those that are particularly high in fiber such as berries, pears, apples, carrots, and leafy greens.

Balanced Meal Compositions

Creating a balanced meal involves more than just choosing the right ingredients; it's about combining them in ways that enhance their digestive benefits:

- **Pairing Fibers with Proteins:** Combine fiber-rich foods with lean proteins to ensure meals are filling and supportive of your digestive system. For example, a chicken salad with mixed greens, nuts, and vinaigrette offers a balanced mix.

- **Small, Frequent Meals:** Eating smaller, more frequent meals can help manage your bile flow more effectively, preventing the overload that can lead to bloating and discomfort.

Gut-Soothing Tactics: Additional Strategies

Beyond diet and meal timing, several lifestyle adjustments and techniques can significantly enhance your digestion and overall comfort. These gut-soothing strategies are designed to complement your dietary changes and provide additional support for managing life without a gallbladder.

Hydration

Keeping well-hydrated is essential for good digestion:

- **Water Intake:** Drink plenty of water throughout the day to help digest food and dissolve nutrients, making them easier to absorb. Aim for at least eight 8-ounce glasses of water daily.

- **Limit Caffeine and Alcohol:** These can irritate the digestive tract and exacerbate symptoms. Moderation is key, and opting for herbal teas can be a soothing alternative.

Exercise

Regular physical activity can help improve digestion and prevent constipation:

- **Gentle Exercise:** Activities like walking, yoga, and light jogging can stimulate the natural contraction of intestinal muscles, helping to move food through your digestive system.

- **Post-Meal Activity:** A gentle walk after meals can encourage digestion and reduce symptoms of bloating and discomfort.

Stress Management

Stress can significantly impact your digestive system:

- **Relaxation Techniques:** Practices such as deep breathing, meditation, and mindfulness can reduce stress and potentially improve your digestive health.

- **Regular Sleep Patterns:** Ensuring you get enough sleep and maintain a regular sleep schedule helps regulate bodily functions, including digestion.

Eating Environment

The environment in which you eat can affect how well you digest your food:

- **Mindful Eating:** Be present during meals, avoid distractions like TV or smartphones, and focus on enjoying your food. This mindfulness can help you chew thoroughly and eat at a slower pace, which is better for digestion.

- **Comfortable Seating:** Sitting comfortably while eating helps your body relax and optimally position itself for digestion.

Herbal Supplements

Certain herbs and supplements are known for their digestive benefits:

- **Ginger:** Known for its anti-inflammatory properties, ginger can help reduce nausea and promote smooth digestion.

- **Peppermint:** Peppermint tea or supplements can soothe the intestines and relieve symptoms like bloating and gas.

- **Probiotics:** These can help maintain healthy gut flora, which is essential for digestion and can be particularly beneficial if you're experiencing symptoms related to small intestine bacterial overgrowth (SIBO).

It's important to consult with a healthcare provider before starting any new supplement to ensure it's safe and appropriate for your specific health situation.

Implementing these gut-soothing tactics into your daily routine can provide significant relief and support for your digestive system. By adopting these additional strategies, you can further enhance your ability to manage a gallbladder-free lifestyle effectively, maintaining comfort and promoting overall digestive health.

Day 1:

- **Breakfast:** Low-Fat Blueberry Yogurt Parfait
- **Snack:** Carrot and Hummus Roll-Ups
- **Lunch:** Grilled Chicken Caesar Salad with Low-Fat Dressing
- **Dinner:** Herb-Roasted Chicken Breast with Steamed Asparagus
- **Dessert:** Baked Apple Cinnamon Oatmeal Cups

Day 2:

- **Breakfast:** Oatmeal Pancakes with Fresh Strawberry Sauce
- **Snack:** Greek Yogurt and Berry Compote
- **Lunch:** Quinoa Tabbouleh with Lemon and Herbs
- **Dinner:** Pork Tenderloin with Apple Cider Reduction
- **Dessert:** Low-Fat Vanilla Yogurt Parfait with Berries and Granola

Day 3:

- **Breakfast:** Scrambled Egg Whites with Spinach and Mushrooms
- **Snack:** Roasted Chickpeas with Sea Salt
- **Lunch:** Turkey and Avocado Wrap with Whole Wheat Tortilla
- **Dinner:** Vegetable Lasagna with Low-Fat Ricotta and Spinach
- **Dessert:** Carrot Cake with Low-Fat Cream Cheese Frosting

Day 4:

- **Breakfast:** Banana Almond Smoothie Bowl
- **Snack:** Avocado and Shrimp Salad Cups
- **Lunch:** Baked Salmon with Dill and Lemon over Greens
- **Dinner:** Grilled Tilapia with Lemon Herb Quinoa
- **Dessert:** Banana Nut Muffins with Whole Wheat

Day 5:

- **Breakfast:** Avocado Toast on Whole Grain Bread
- **Snack:** Vegetable Spring Rolls with Peanut Dipping Sauce
- **Lunch:** Chicken and Vegetable Stir-Fry with Ginger Sauce
- **Dinner:** Beef Stir-Fry with Broccoli and Bell Pepper
- **Dessert:** Chocolate-Dipped Strawberries with Dark Chocolate

Day 6:

- **Breakfast:** Turkey Bacon and Egg White Muffins
- **Snack:** Baked Apple Chips
- **Lunch:** Pasta Primavera with Olive Oil and Parmesan
- **Dinner:** Butternut Squash Risotto
- **Dessert:** Almond and Date Energy Balls

Day 7:

- **Breakfast:** Overnight Chia Pudding with Kiwi and Mango

- **Snack:** Mozzarella and Tomato Basil Bruschetta
- **Lunch:** Turkey Meatballs in Marinara Sauce over Spaghetti Squash
- **Dinner:** Shrimp Scampi over Whole Wheat Pasta
- **Dessert:** Coconut Water Fruit Popsicles

Day 8:

- **Breakfast:** Quinoa Porridge with Honey and Almonds
- **Snack:** Cucumber and Turkey Mini Sandwiches
- **Lunch:** Roasted Beet and Goat Cheese Salad
- **Dinner:** Turkey Meatloaf with Sweet Potato Mash
- **Dessert:** Poached Pears with Cinnamon and Clove

Day 9:

- **Breakfast:** Cottage Cheese and Pineapple Bowl
- **Snack:** Spiced Pumpkin Seeds
- **Lunch:** Vegetable and Bean Chili
- **Dinner:** Vegetarian Paella with Saffron and Mixed Vegetables
- **Dessert:** Raspberry Chia Seed Pudding

Day 10:

- **Breakfast:** Multigrain French Toast with Agave Syrup
- **Snack:** Hard-Boiled Egg and Avocado Bowl
- **Lunch:** Baked Tilapia with Mango Salsa
- **Dinner:** Stuffed Bell Peppers with Ground Turkey and Farro

- **Dessert:** Baked Peaches with Honey and Almonds

Day 11:

- **Breakfast:** Smoked Salmon and Cream Cheese on a Bagel Thin
- **Snack:** Sweet Potato and Black Bean Quesadillas
- **Lunch:** Asian Chicken Salad with Low-Sodium Soy Dressing
- **Dinner:** Salmon Burgers with Avocado Salsa
- **Dessert:** Mango and Sticky Rice

Day 12:

- **Breakfast:** Berry and Greek Yogurt Smoothie
- **Snack:** Tuna Salad Stuffed Tomatoes
- **Lunch:** Stuffed Acorn Squash with Quinoa and Cranberries
- **Dinner:** Roasted Duck with Orange Glaze
- **Dessert:** Blueberry Lemon Zest Muffins

Day 13:

- **Breakfast:** Baked Sweet Potato and Kale Hash
- **Snack:** Chicken Lettuce Wraps with Mango Salsa
- **Lunch:** Southwest Chicken Bowl with Brown Rice and Black Beans
- **Dinner:** Spaghetti with Turkey Bolognese Sauce
- **Dessert:** Flourless Chocolate Cake with Raspberry Sauce

Day 14:

- **Breakfast:** Apple and Walnut Yogurt Parfait
- **Snack:** Broccoli and Cheese Mini Quiches

- **Lunch:** Mediterranean Tuna Salad with Mixed Greens
- **Dinner:** Beef and Vegetable Kabobs with Yogurt Sauce
- **Dessert:** Low-Fat Cheesecake with Fresh Fruit Topping

Day 15:

- **Breakfast:** Low-Fat Cottage Cheese Pancakes
- **Snack:** Kale Chips with Nutritional Yeast
- **Lunch:** Broccoli and Cheese Stuffed Chicken Breast
- **Dinner:** Lamb Chops with Mint Pesto
- **Dessert:** Kiwi and Pineapple Fruit Tart

Day 16:

- **Breakfast:** Apple and Walnut Yogurt Parfait
- **Snack:** Vegetable Spring Rolls with Peanut Dipping Sauce
- **Lunch:** Roasted Cauliflower Soup with Low-Fat Cream
- **Dinner:** Baked Trout with Walnut Crust
- **Dessert:** No-Bake Peanut Butter Cookies

Day 17:

- **Breakfast:** Multigrain French Toast with Agave Syrup
- **Snack:** Roasted Chickpeas with Sea Salt
- **Lunch:** Vegan Curry with Tofu and Vegetables
- **Dinner:** Moroccan Chicken with Olives and Lemons
- **Dessert:** Coconut Water Fruit Popsicles

Day 18:

- **Breakfast:** Berry and Greek Yogurt Smoothie
- **Snack:** Edamame and Cranberry Salad
- **Lunch:** Lentil Soup with Carrots and Celery
- **Dinner:** Vegetarian Paella with Saffron and Mixed Vegetables
- **Dessert:** Baked Apple Cinnamon Oatmeal Cups

Day 19:

- **Breakfast:** Quinoa Porridge with Honey and Almonds
- **Snack:** Avocado and Shrimp Salad Cups
- **Lunch:** Vegetarian Stuffed Peppers with Brown Rice
- **Dinner:** Ratatouille with Eggplant, Zucchini, and Tomato
- **Dessert:** Low-Fat Vanilla Yogurt Parfait with Berries and Granola

Day 20:

- **Breakfast:** Scrambled Egg Whites with Spinach and Mushrooms
- **Snack:** Baked Apple Chips
- **Lunch:** Chicken and Vegetable Stir-Fry with Ginger Sauce
- **Dinner:** Roasted Duck with Orange Glaze
- **Dessert:** Lemon Angel Food Cake

Day 21:

- **Breakfast:** Banana Almond Smoothie Bowl
- **Snack:** Greek Yogurt and Berry Compote
- **Lunch:** Chickpea Salad with Cucumber and Feta
- **Dinner:** Beef Stir-Fry with Broccoli and Bell Pepper

- **Dessert:** Carrot Cake with Low-Fat Cream Cheese Frosting

Day 22:

- **Breakfast:** Overnight Chia Pudding with Kiwi and Mango
- **Snack:** Cucumber and Turkey Mini Sandwiches
- **Lunch:** Pasta Primavera with Olive Oil and Parmesan
- **Dinner:** Grilled Tilapia with Lemon Herb Quinoa
- **Dessert:** Peach and Ginger Sorbet

Day 23:

- **Breakfast:** Avocado Toast on Whole Grain Bread
- **Snack:** Caprese Salad Skewers with Balsamic Glaze
- **Lunch:** Turkey Meatballs in Marinara Sauce over Spaghetti Squash
- **Dinner:** Shrimp Scampi over Whole Wheat Pasta
- **Dessert:** Pumpkin Spice Rice Pudding

Day 24:

- **Breakfast:** Turkey Bacon and Egg White Muffins
- **Snack:** Sweet Potato and Black Bean Quesadillas
- **Lunch:** Baked Tilapia with Mango Salsa
- **Dinner:** Chicken Parmesan with Low-Fat Mozzarella
- **Dessert:** Banana Nut Muffins with Whole Wheat

Day 25:

- **Breakfast:** Baked Sweet Potato and Kale Hash
- **Snack:** Tuna Salad Stuffed Tomatoes
- **Lunch:** Stuffed Acorn Squash with Quinoa and Cranberries
- **Dinner:** Stuffed Bell Peppers with Ground Turkey and Farro
- **Dessert:** Chocolate-Dipped Strawberries with Dark Chocolate

Day 26:

- **Breakfast:** Smoked Salmon and Cream Cheese on a Bagel Thin
- **Snack:** Broccoli and Cheese Mini Quiches
- **Lunch:** Southwest Chicken Bowl with Brown Rice and Black Beans
- **Dinner:** Salmon Burgers with Avocado Salsa
- **Dessert:** Almond and Date Energy Balls

Day 27:

- **Breakfast:** Cottage Cheese and Pineapple Bowl
- **Snack:** Chicken Lettuce Wraps with Mango Salsa
- **Lunch:** Mediterranean Tuna Salad with Mixed Greens
- **Dinner:** Beef and Vegetable Kabobs with Yogurt Sauce
- **Dessert:** Baked Peaches with Honey and Almonds

Day 28:

- **Breakfast:** Low-Fat Cottage Cheese Pancakes
- **Snack:** Mozzarella and Tomato Basil Bruschetta
- **Lunch:** Asian Chicken Salad with Low-Sodium Soy Dressing

- **Dinner:** Herb-Roasted Chicken Breast with Steamed Asparagus

- **Dessert:** Low-Fat Cheesecake with Fresh Fruit Topping

Glossary of Terms

Bile: A digestive fluid produced by the liver, stored in the gallbladder, and released into the small intestine to help digest fats. After gallbladder removal, bile flows directly from the liver into the small intestine.

Cholecystectomy: The surgical removal of the gallbladder. This procedure is often performed due to gallstones, inflammation, or other gallbladder-related issues.

Digestive Enzymes: Proteins produced by the digestive system to break down food into nutrients that the body can absorb. Key enzymes include lipase (fats), protease (proteins), and amylase (carbohydrates).

Fat-Soluble Vitamins: Vitamins that are absorbed along with fats in the diet and can be stored in the body's fatty tissue. These include Vitamins A, D, E, and K.

Gallstones: Hard particles that form in the gallbladder, typically consisting of cholesterol or bilirubin, which can cause pain and block bile flow.

Low-Fat Diet: A diet that limits the amount of fat, especially saturated fat and cholesterol. This type of diet is often recommended for individuals without a gallbladder to ease digestion and reduce symptoms.

Micronutrients: Vitamins and minerals required by the body in small amounts for various functions, including maintaining energy levels, improving brain function, and repairing cellular damage.

Macronutrients: The three primary types of nutrients used by the body: carbohydrates, proteins, and fats. They are the main sources of energy for the body.

Probiotics: Live bacteria and yeasts that are beneficial for the digestive system. Probiotics are often called "good" or "helpful" bacteria because they help keep the gut healthy.

SIBO (Small Intestine Bacterial Overgrowth): A condition in which an abnormal amount of bacteria grows in the small intestine, often resulting in symptoms like pain, bloating, and diarrhea, especially common in people without a gallbladder.

Soluble Fiber: A type of fiber that dissolves in water to form a gel-like material. It can help lower blood cholesterol and glucose levels. Soluble fiber is found in oats, peas, beans, apples, citrus fruits, carrots, barley, and psyllium.

Insoluble Fiber: Fiber that does not dissolve in water. It helps move material through the digestive system and increases stool bulk, beneficial for those who struggle with constipation. Common sources include whole wheat flour, wheat bran, nuts, beans, and vegetables.

Appreciation and Bonus Downloads

Dear Reader,

Thank you for trusting me with your dietary journey following gallbladder removal. I hope that this guide serves not only as a tool but as a companion on your path to better health and well-being.

As a token of my appreciation for your commitment to enhancing your lifestyle, I am pleased to offer you exclusive access to two specially designed bonuses.

Gallbladder Diet Mastery Series:
Unlock access to the exclusive email newsletter that provides expert guidance on managing your post-gallbladder diet. This series covers everything from balancing nutrients to simplifying meal preparation, all tailored to help you manage symptoms effectively and make confident dietary choices.

Daily Digest Tracker:
Take control of your diet with this comprehensive journal designed to help you monitor how different foods affect your body. Track your daily intake, note any reactions, and adjust your eating habits to minimize discomfort and optimize health.

Please scan the QR code below to download your bonuses:

Or copy and paste the URL:

https://qrco.de/bf7rHd

Thank you once again for choosing this guide. For more resources and future publications, don't forget to follow my author page.

Wishing you health and happiness,

Ada Bennett

www.ingramcontent.com/pod-product-compliance
Lightning Source LLC
Chambersburg PA
CBHW081843250726
48659CB00008B/2583